**Exposure of
the Pregnant Patient
to Diagnostic
Radiations**

J. B. Lippincott Company
Philadelphia

London
Mexico City
New York
St. Louis
São Paulo
Sydney

Exposure of the Pregnant Patient to Diagnostic Radiations

A Guide to Medical Management

Louis K. Wagner, Ph.D.

Associate Professor
Department of Radiology
University of Texas Medical School at Houston
Houston, Texas

Richard G. Lester, M.D.

Dean, Vice-President for Academic Affairs
Professor of Radiology
Eastern Virginia Medical School
Norfolk, Virginia

Luis R. Saldana, M.D.

Clinical Associate Professor
Department of Obstetrics and Gynecology
University of Cincinnati Medical Center;
Director, Division of Maternal–Fetal Medicine
Academic Director for Obstetrics
Department of Obstetrics and Gynecology
Bethesda Hospital
Cincinnati, Ohio

Acquisitions Editor: William Burgower
Sponsoring Editor: Richard Winters
Manuscript Editor: Helen Ewan
Indexer: Sandra King
Design Director: Tracy Baldwin
Design Coordinator: Earl Gerhart
Designer: Arlene Putterman
Production Supervisor: Kathleen P. Dunn
Production Assistant: Susan Hess
Composition: International Computaprint
  Corporation
Printer/Binder: R. R. Donnelly & Sons Company

6 5 4 3 2 1

Library of Congress Cataloging in Publication Data

Wagner, Louis K.
Exposure of the Pregnant patient to diagnostic
radiations.

    Includes bibliographies and index.
    1. Fetus—Effect of radiation on. 2. Pregnant
women—Radiography. 3. Radiation—Dosage. I.
Lester, Richard G. II. Saldana, Luis R. III. Title.
[DNLM: 1. Fetus—radiation effects. 2. Pregnancy
—radiation effects. 3. Radiography—adverse
effects. 4. Radiography—in pregnancy.
WQ 202 W133e]
RG627.6.R33W34   1985   618.3′20757
84-27807
ISBN 0-397-50667-8

*Dedicated
to the memory of
John Kenneth Cotten Wagner*

Preface

The diagnostic radiological management of pregnant or potentially pregnant patients is a major concern of physicians because of possibly adverse effects that radiation may have on unborn children. This book developed from the need perceived by the authors for a reference source that cohesively addresses the patient management issues posed by this problem. The authors have designed *Exposure of the Pregnant Patient to Diagnostic Radiations: A Guide to Medical Management* for use by both obstetricians and general practitioners, as well as radiologists and medical physicists, so that it can serve as a useful guide in a busy clinical setting.

The referring physician and the radiologist share responsibility in the diagnostic evaluation of fertile women. Just as caution should be exercised when prescribing certain drugs to pregnant or possibly pregnant patients, care also should be exercised when referring these patients for diagnostic radiological study.

The patient usually identifies "her doctor," the referring physician, as the one providing care and whose counsel is the most important to her. The referring physician should not only investigate the possibility of pregnancy but should also understand and relate to the patient the degree to which a diagnostic study might compromise the pregnancy. The text and flowcharts are designed to assist in making benefit–risk decisions.

Consultants, although highly regarded by the referring physician, do not always have the time to establish personal rapport with the patient. This relationship is the bedrock of effective counseling. It is, therefore, important that the primary-care physician effectively communicate a consultant's opinion. Methods of presenting data and communicating risks to a patient are reviewed.

Radiologists are ultimately responsible for their delivery of radiation to patients. The radiologist should be notified of the potential for pregnancy and, in some cases, should be involved in the counseling prior to the diagnostic study. They should be able to place the benefits of a study and the associated risks into perspective for the primary-care physician and the patient. They should also be able to make decisions about how to minimize any potential radiation exposure to a conceptus. Radiologists will find this text helpful in providing counsel. They will also find much of the discussion directly and practically applicable to them. For example, some suggestions of how to modify studies or otherwise reduce conceptus dose are included. Radiologists' role in investigating possible pregnancy is also discussed.

Physicists are often consulted on the techniques that can be employed to minimize radiation dose to a patient and are asked to calculate either the anticipated or the delivered conceptus dose. We review not only standard methods for achieving these goals, but also point out subtle aspects of the problem and potential sources of error.

Part I of the book provides the necessary background for an in-depth understanding of the diagnostic radiations used and the risks they pose to unborn children. X-ray imaging, radionuclide studies, ultrasound examinations, and magnetic resonance are all reviewed. The reader need not refer to this material when applying the flow charts to the clinical setting. However, we recommend that the reader study Part I, as well as the chapters containing the flow charts, *prior* to being confronted with a clinical situation. The physician will then be well-prepared when a decision on management of a patient is needed. This may avert unnecessary anxiety and alarm.

Part II addresses the situation in which a pregnant or potentially pregnant woman may need a radiological examination. The text and flowcharts guide the reader in collecting the necessary data, in weighing the potential benefits of an examination against the concomitant risks of prenatal irradiation, and in counseling the patient.

Part III considers the management of a patient who has received a radiological examination and who is *post facto* discovered to have been pregnant at the time. Patient care is discussed in terms of counseling, data collection, risk evaluation, and decisions about the future of the pregnancy.

For the sake of completeness, Appendices A and B review the calculational techniques that can be used to estimate absorbed dose to a conceptus from x-ray or radionuclide studies. The authors do not anticipate that these sections will be useful to everyone using the text. Those readers trained in radiological physics may find the data and the equations helpful.

Examples are used to describe their proper application and their associated pitfalls.

For clarity, it is necessary to adopt strict definitions for certain terms used frequently throughout the text. In available reference material, the terms embryo, fetus, and embryo/fetus are most frequently used when describing prenatal development. We have attempted to adhere to their strict definitions. *Embryo* refers to the prenatal offspring during its most rapid development. This occurs in the human during the second through seventh weeks after fertilization. *Fetus* refers to the unborn offspring from the eighth week after fertilization until birth. The term *embryo/fetus* combines these two stages of development. The term *conceptus* is used to describe all the prenatal tissues from the moment of conception until birth.

Likewise, strict definitions to describe the age of the conceptus have been adopted. In this text, three terms are used: gestation age, conception age, and menstrual age. *Gestation age* is used generally to describe the maturity of the conceptus without any specific reference to the time elapsed since fertilization. For example, we could make the statement that "radiation risk to a conceptus depends strongly on the gestation age." *Conception age* refers to the time elapsed since the moment of conception. For instance, "The conception age was 3 weeks." *Menstrual age* refers to the time elapsed since the last menstrual period. In the previous example, the menstrual age would usually be about 5 weeks.

The authors are grateful for the numerous contributions from individuals whose only recognition is a mention of their names in the preface. This is a meager and inadequate compensation for their generous and excellent work. We thank Barbara Cook, Jorene Jones-York, and Kathy Norred for typing the initial drafts of the text. Special thanks are extended to Sandee Sundve for typing multiple revisions. We extend our gratitude to Dye Jensen for his assistance in translating foreign articles, to Roz Vecchio and Lew Hondros for their photographic work, and to Phyllis Love and David Dohanyos for preparing the illustrations.

Several people rendered significant recommendations for improving the text. Benjamin Archer, Viren Balsara, Berel Held, Martin Graham, and Lawrence Rothenberg provided valuable commentary. The recommendations from Fred Kremkau, Jonathan Ophir, Paul Murphy, E. Edmund Kim, Jean Delayre, Stewart Bushong, and Gary Barnes have resulted in a greatly improved text and are sincerely appreciated. We especially thank William J. Schull, Joel Gray, Harris Jackson, and Ed McCullough for their meticulous and perspicacious reviews. All have contributed in significant and important ways to the development of this text.

Contents

**Exposure of
the Pregnant Patient
to Diagnostic
Radiations**

Introduction

The following vignette illustrates how diagnostic radiologic studies can rapidly complicate a simple diagnosis of pregnancy.

> The tests have been completed and you've called in your patient. "Well, Mrs. Adams," you begin. "It's really quite simple, you're pregnant, about two and a half months."
>
> Mrs. Adams smiles, and then becomes anxious. "Doctor, you remember when I went to the emergency room last month because of the pain in my back? Remember? They took kidney x rays, lots of them! And chest x rays too. Aren't x rays dangerous for my baby? What will happen to my baby?"

Mrs. Adams's circumstance occurs infrequently, but it is not exceptional. Nor is the situation exceptional where a woman, known to be pregnant, needs radiologic study for a health problem. In each case, the physician should advise and counsel the patient regarding the risks of radiation. If she is to receive a radiologic study, the risks should be compared to the potential benefits for her and her child.

This book is designed to provide the physician with a knowledge about radiations used in diagnostic radiologic procedures, an understanding of the radiologic data needed to assess the risks for pregnant women, information on the known risks for unborn children, and guidelines to manage and counsel women and their families. It outlines the decisions to be made when a woman, already exposed to radiation, is discovered to be pregnant, or when a pregnant woman has medical problems that require diagnostic examination using x rays, radioisotopes, ultrasound, or magnetic resonance.

Diagnostic examinations in pregnant women should be performed only when there is sufficient reason to believe the benefit to her or her child, or to both, exceeds the known or reasonably suspected risks. These trade-offs are often perceived as a dilemma. Some of the data are controversial and incomplete. The issues are emotionally sensitive for both prospective parents and physicians. Although many publications have addressed the biologic effects of radiation on conceptuses, there has not been an easily accessible, comprehensive reference source that addresses the patient-oriented issues encountered by the practitioner.

The availability of data on biologic effects does not, by itself, make the data readily useful. It is often difficult to assess risk from technical data, and still more difficult to place the risk into a perspective from which an informed decision can be made. For example, the carcinogenic risk of x rays on the unborn is often expressed in relative terms by comparing the postnatal cancer incidence in exposed and unexposed populations, or by stating the radiocarcinogenic sensitivity of the unborn relative to that of an adult. These factors may perceptually exaggerate the actual risk that the child will develop cancer.

To illustrate this point, consider the following. Data suggest that childhood cancer is increased by 250% for children who receive 1 rad* during the first trimester (BEIR Committee, (1980). The relative risk factor is 3.5 (*i.e.*, [250% + 100%]/100% = 3.5) when compared with children who received no diagnostic radiation. These same data also suggest that the early conceptus is about 16 times more sensitive to radiocarcinogenic x rays than are adults. Both these statements are equally valid, and both are uninformative without knowing the normal incidence of childhood cancer or how sensitive adults are to the carcinogenic effect of x rays.

If the normal incidence of childhood cancer were 2 cases for every 10 children, 80% of all children would *not* develop cancer. A 3.5-times increase in cancer risk would be catastrophic, because 70% of the children receiving 1 rad would develop cancer and only 30% would not. In that setting, the benefit of diagnostic examinations to pregnant women would be severely compromised by the risk of radiation-induced childhood cancer.

The actual incidence of childhood cancer is about 1 in 1500. This means that 99.93% of all unexposed children do not develop cancer. Assuming a 250% increase in relative risk per rad if radiation is received in the first trimester, 2.5 additional cases of childhood cancer might result. If 1 rad is de-

---

*The rad is a unit of absorbed dose of ionizing radiation (See Chap. 2). It is defined as an energy transfer of 100 ergs per gram of tissue. One rad is a typical conceptus dose from several lower abdominal radiographs.

livered to 1500 nonpregnant adults, only 0.15 of these adults would be expected to develop radiation-induced cancer. Therefore, an early conceptus is about 16 times more radiosensitive to the carcinogenic effects of x-rays than are adults (2.5 ÷ 0.15 ≃ 16). Even so, in absolute terms the risk of radiation-induced childhood cancer is still quite small because the likelihood of *not* developing cancer following a 1-rad dose would be 99.77% (1496.5 healthy children out of 1500 exposed to 1 rad *in utero*). The perspective of risk from the counseling physician's and the patient's point-of-view is considerably different depending on how the data are presented. The physician must decide if the expected benefit to the mother or the conceptus outweighs the potential risk and then appropriately counsel the patient.

Furthermore, conception age plays a significant role in risk evaluation. For the second or third trimester, the assumed increase in relative risk of childhood cancer is 64% per rad. Using the above example, this means the likelihood of not developing cancer after a 1-rad conceptus dose is 99.89%, an 0.04% reduction from the normal incidence. (The reader is cautioned that, as noted in Chap. 4, these risk factors are controversial, and an actual causal link between *in utero* radiation and childhood cancer is debatable.)

Risks associated with radiation depend critically on two factors: conception age and the amount of radiation delivered. During some stages of gestation, the risks involved are so small and so uncertain that the amount of radiation delivered from most diagnostic studies is inconsequential to patient management. During other stages of gestation, a lack of perspective regarding the levels of conceptus irradiation from diagnostic radiologic procedures often leads to an exaggeration of the risks. Many radiographic examinations deliver very little radiation to the conceptus, frequently much less than all the radiation the conceptus will receive from naturally occurring environmental radiation. In this situation, the risks from medical irradiation are negligible and irrelevant to proper medical care.

On the other hand, there are circumstances where the amount of radiation and the conception age are both critical to patient management. This would be the case for diagnostic evaluation of the lower abdomen of a patient whose conceptus is at a stage known to be sensitive to radiation-induced mental retardation. In these circumstances, a radiation dose evaluation is necessary, and this usually requires the assistance of a radiological physicist. An estimation of conceptus dose from abdominal examinations depends on the radiation output of the equipment used, the sensitivity of the image recorder (usually film), the size of the patient, and a number of other technical factors. Such data are usually available, although not always readily accessible. Physicians should not rely on guesses or simple estimates to acquire such information in critical circumstances. Reliable estimates should be obtained from personnel trained in dosimetry.

In subsequent chapters, the scientific literature is summarized in a perspective from which physicians can make knowledgeable decisions regarding the proper handling of the pregnant or possibly pregnant patient. If the scientific data are controversial, the problem is addressed in light of this controversy. We recognize that there is still much to learn regarding radiation effects on the unborn. This sometimes makes risk analysis difficult. However, it is irresponsible to permit the unknown to push us into rash and drastic actions. To the contrary, it is reasonable to assess the facts, admit our ignorance regarding questions we cannot answer, contemplate the consequences in light of what we do know, and then act in the best interest of the patient and the conceptus.

Part I of the text reviews some elementary radiobiology and physics of diagnostic radiations from x-ray, nuclear, ultrasound, and magnetic resonance studies. Misconceptions about the amount of diagnostic radiation, as well as about the interactions of radiation in tissues, often contribute to overblown conclusions regarding the risks involved. Conversely, ignorance about these same matters may lead to a false sense of security regarding the safety of diagnostic studies. Just as physicians should be aware of possible side-effects of drugs and have knowledge of their metabolism, so, too, physicians should understand what radiation is and how it interacts in humans. These chapters provide the physician with information applicable to the pregnant patient.

Part II discusses the management of pregnant patients who need radiologic evaluation. Part III reviews the *post facto* management of patients who were not known to be pregnant when a radiologic procedure was done. The management issues are summarized in the flowcharts at the beginning of each of these sections. These flowcharts outline the questions each physician should address when referring a potentially pregnant patient for a radiologic, radiopharmaceutical, ultrasonic, or magnetic resonance study, or when considering the care of a patient who is discovered to have been pregnant at the time an ionizing radiation study was performed.

Reference

BEIR Committee (Committee on the Biological Effects of Ionizing Radiations): The Effects on Populations to Exposure to Low Levels of Ionizing Radiation: 1980, p 450. Washington, DC, National Academy Press, 1980

Part I
Diagnostic Radiations and Risks to Unborn Children

This section provides background to understand what radiation is, how it is used for diagnoses, why it can have deleterious effects on a conceptus, and what the possible consequences might be. Although necessary for an in-depth comprehension of the subject, it is not necessary to read when applying the guidelines of Parts II or III. Reference is made to information in Part I when needed. We do recommend that the reader review this section before being confronted with a pregnant patient who needs or has had diagnostic studies. A knowledgeable background aids in the immediate counseling of these patients. Part II gives guidelines on the management of a pregnant patient who needs a radiologic study. For management of patients already exposed to radiation while pregnant, see Part III.

Chapter 1
The Diagnostic
Radiations
and Their Mechanisms
for Injury

Diagnostic radiologic modalities include x-ray radiography, radionuclide studies, ultrasound, and magnetic resonance. Radiographic x rays are machine-generated, externally administered ionizing radiations. The ionizing radiations from radionuclide studies emanate from substances that are internally introduced into the patient. Ultrasound uses machine-generated nonionizing sonic waves. Magnetic resonance employs static and time-dependent magnetic fields as well as radiofrequency waves. This chapter reviews, under separate headings, the radiations of each modality, their uses in medicine, and their mechanisms for producing biologic effects.

Ionizing Radiations

DIAGNOSTIC X RAYS

Diagnostic x radiation is ubiquitous in modern medical care. Radiographic studies such as the chest examination, fluoroscopic studies such as the upper gastrointestinal series, and technically complex evaluations such as computed tomography (CT), digital radiography, and selective arteriography all make use of x rays.

Visible light and x radiation are similar in that both are composed of packets of pure energy that travel in straight lines at the speed of light and have no mass or charge. These energy packets are called *photons*. Just as

7

light is electronically generated in a light bulb by flipping a switch, so too, x rays can be turned on and off with a switch. X rays exist for only a brief moment while the switch is on. The duration is usually less than 1 second for the standard radiograph. After this, the patient does not retain or emit any radiation.

X rays used in diagnostic radiology differ from visible light photons in that they are tens of thousands of times more energetic. The energy of a light photon is a few electron volts (eV). (An electron volt is a very small unit of energy equivalent to 1.6×10^{-19} joules or 4.4×10^{-26} kilowatt hours.) Diagnostic x rays range in energy from 10 to 150 kiloelectron volts (keV).

Because of their energy, x rays entering a patient's abdomen have a finite chance of passing through the entire tissue space without colliding (interacting) with any of the electrons or atoms in the patient. Those photons that successfully traverse the patient create the radiographic image. However, most x rays collide with electrons in the patient's tissues before completely penetrating the abdomen.

The probability of interaction increases as the amount of material in the path of the x ray increases and as the atomic weight of its elemental composition increases. Figure 1-1 demonstrates this principle in a chest radiograph. Dark areas of an x-ray film result when high intensities of x rays strike the film. Transparent areas appear when the x rays are very low in intensity. In creating a chest radiograph, many x rays pass through the lung where the likelihood of interaction with an electron is relatively small. This is because the lung space is occupied by a large amount of air, and so the amount of tissue that x rays traverse is significantly less here than in the mediastinum. The air-filled lung, therefore, appears dark on the film. On the other hand, x rays passing through the mediastinum must traverse not only a large amount of soft tissue, but also the calcium-rich vertebrae. X rays in this area of the thorax have a much smaller chance of passing through the entire patient thickness. This area of the film is therefore exposed to only a very few x rays and appears almost transparent on the film. In summary, the radiograph is a photographic record of the elemental composition and amount of matter that x rays had to traverse before reaching the film.

X rays that collide with atoms or electrons transfer all or part of their energy. When atoms of molecules absorb x ray energy, electrons break away from their molecular orbits, creating excited or ionized molecules within the patient—thus the term *ionizing* radiation. When these electrons are propelled from their bound molecular states by x rays, they eject other electrons. This creates further ionization or excitation of other molecules in the body until all the energy imparted to the initial electrons is absorbed by the tissue.

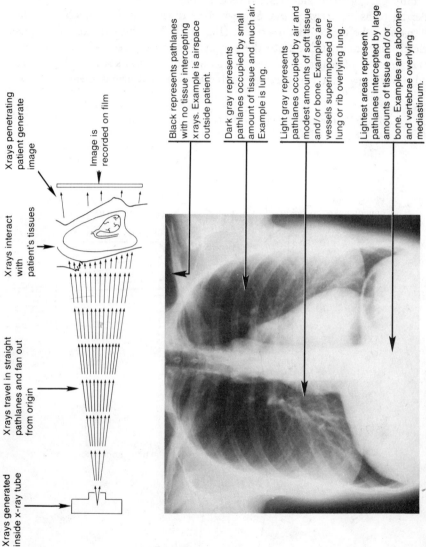

Xrays penetrating patient generate image

Image is recorded on film

Xrays interact with patient's tissues

Xrays travel in straight pathlanes and fan out from origin

Xrays generated inside x-ray tube

Black represents pathlanes with no tissue intercepting xrays. Example is airspace outside patient.

Dark gray represents pathlanes occupied by small amount of tissue and much air. Example is lung.

Light gray represents pathlanes occupied by air and modest amounts of soft tissue and/or bone. Examples are vessels superimposed over lung or rib overlying lung.

Lightest areas represent pathlanes intercepted by large amounts of tissue and/or bone. Examples are abdomen and vertebrae overlying mediastinum.

FIG. 1-1. The making of a radiograph.

Radiation effects in diagnostic radiology are confined primarily to the tissues directly exposed to the x-ray beam. In a chest radiograph, the radiation is confined primarily to the thorax. Those x rays that give up all their energy are "absorbed" by the tissue and no longer exist. X rays that give up only part of their energy are diverted from their line of travel. These are referred to as *scattered x rays.* Some will be diverted in the direction of the uterus and the conceptus, if present (Fig. 1-2). For chest radiography, any deleterious radiation effects to the conceptus can only result from this very small amount of scattered x rays as well as from x rays scattered by the air and a very few that penetrate through the protective encasement of the x-

FIG. 1-2. The chest radiograph and conceptus irradiation.

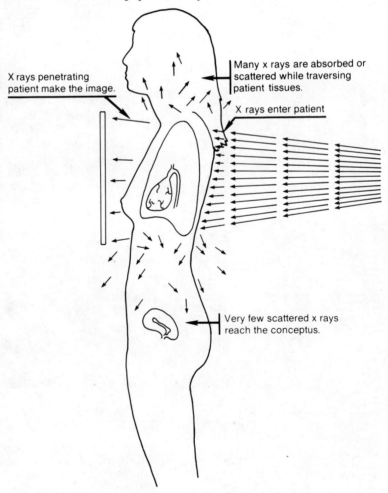

ray tube. These latter x rays are referred to as *leakage radiation*. In a typical setting, about 200 posteroanterior and lateral chest radiographs would be required to deliver to the conceptus an amount of radiation equal to that received during gestation from cosmic rays and naturally existing radioactive matter, like carbon 14, present in organic food supplies.

Diagnostic examinations involving the pelvis, such as kidney–ureter–bladder or a barium enema, directly irradiate the conceptus (Fig. 1-3). In

FIG. 1-3. The abdominal radiograph and conceptus irradiation.

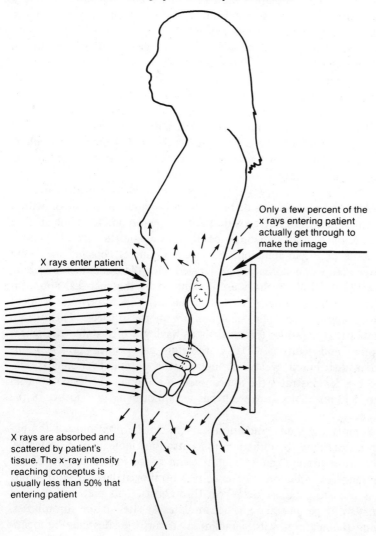

Only a few percent of the x rays entering patient actually get through to make the image

X rays enter patient

X rays are absorbed and scattered by patient's tissue. The x-ray intensity reaching conceptus is usually less than 50% that entering patient

this case the conceptus receives a higher level of radiation (typically two to five times more per film than all the natural background radiation received during gestation). This represents a greater risk for biologic effect than does a chest radiograph. Although this risk is usually small, it may, in some cases, be substantial. The actual risk depends on many factors, which are discussed in Chapters 4 and 6.

RADIONUCLIDE EXAMINATIONS

Atomic nuclei that emit radiation are called *radioactive nuclides,* or simply *radionuclides.* Studies using these substances differ significantly from x-ray examinations. Radionuclides usually act as labels on pharmacologic agents, although they sometimes act alone as self-labeled agents. The labeled agents are called *radiopharmaceuticals.* They are typically injected intravenously (although for some purposes agents are given *per os* or in other fashions). After a radiopharmaceutical is administered, it is distributed by physiologic and metabolic mechanisms, and radiation emanates from within the patient. The radiation continues to emanate from the patient's organs for a period of time, from many minutes to a few months depending on the radiopharmaceutical used. These substances may be used for either imaging or nonimaging diagnostic purposes.

For an imaging study, a radiation detector is used to provide a map or picture of how the radiation is distributed throughout an organ or within the body. The image does not provide the high-quality anatomic detail that x-ray films do, but it may sometimes be of more diagnostic value because it evaluates tissue or organ function. A typical example, depicted in Figure 1-4, is a liver scan using sulfur colloid labeled with the radionuclide technetium 99m (^{99m}Tc). (Radionuclides are designated by the chemical abbreviation of their associated atom [Tc = technetium] and by a number identifying how many protons plus neutrons are in the nucleus. The *m* is a special symbol that identifies this nucleus as having a metastable configuration of protons and neutrons. ^{99m}Tc is therefore an "isomer" of ^{99}Tc.) Sulfur colloid is distributed evenly throughout the normal liver and spleen, and Figure 1-4 demonstrates the appearance of a lesion. The lesion appears as a deficit of radioactivity because it has an abnormally low uptake of the radiopharmaceutical.

For a nonimaging study, radiation sensors can be used outside the patient to probe anatomy for radiation concentrations indicative of problems, or blood or urine samples can be acquired and tested for the normal or abnormal presence of radiation. For example, fibrinogen labeled with iodine 125 (^{125}I) is used to diagnose deep-vein thrombosis. This material, injected into an unaffected peripheral vein, accumulates at sites of the thromboses. By surveying the anatomy with a radiation sensor, the sites may be identi-

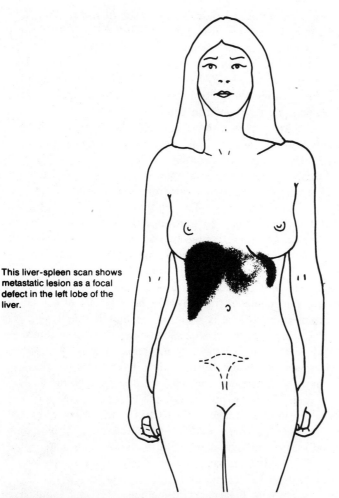

This liver-spleen scan shows metastatic lesion as a focal defect in the left lobe of the liver.

FIG. 1-4. Radionuclide scan of a woman's liver and spleen.

fied. Another example is the use of phosphorus 32 (^{32}P) to investigate phosphorus uptake in the eye. Abnormal concentrations indicate the presence of melanoma. An example of a study that analyzes activity in urine samples is the Schilling test to diagnose pernicious anemia. In this case two pharmaceuticals, vitamin B intrinsic-factor complex and vitamin B, are labeled with the respective radionuclides cobalt 57 (^{57}Co) and cobalt 58 (^{58}Co). These two radionuclides are distinguished by the energies of their respective radiations, specifically 122 keV photons for ^{57}Co versus 811 keV photons for ^{58}Co. The relative excretion of these two radionuclides in the urine produces the required diagnostic information.

Gamma radiation is the principal radiation used for *in vivo* radionuclide studies. Like x rays, gamma rays are also photons. They differ in that gamma rays generally originate from the nucleus of an atom* and are usually more energetic than diagnostic x rays. Gamma rays currently used in medical imaging have energies from 81 keV to 511 keV. The most frequently used energy is 140 keV. Nonimaging radionuclide studies use gamma rays with energies up to about 1.3 megaelectron volts (MeV).

Because gamma rays are generally more energetic than x rays, they penetrate tissue more readily. Like x rays, gamma rays will interact with atoms and electrons in the body and cause ionization.

Other radiations can also be emitted by radioactive atoms. Agents used in nuclear medicine might emit electrons, positrons (the positively charged counterpart to an electron), and x rays. The emitted electrons or positrons are collectively called *beta particles*. In addition, the orbital electrons of many radioactive atoms can become excited by nuclear emissions. This may result in subsequent emission of electrons and x rays from atomic orbits.

Beta particles provide no imaging information and usually travel only about a millimeter in tissue. One nonimaging diagnostic use of beta particles is the ^{32}P test for melanoma of the eye. Beta particles are also used in positron emission tomography. This is a technique that indirectly utilizes positrons for imaging. Although the positrons provide no imaging information themselves, they react with electrons in an interesting way. A positron is attracted to electrons in matter because they have opposite charges. When a positron collides with an electron, the two destroy each other. This mutual annihilation gives rise to two photons, each having an energy of 511 keV. These photons are used to image the activity inside the body. Except for these and a few other uses, beta particles are untoward by-products of radioactivity that only cause biologic damage through ionization and excitation. Some radionuclides emit beta particles; others do not. An example of a radionuclide that emits both gamma and beta rays is Iodine 131 (^{131}I). Radionuclides that do not emit beta particles include ^{99m}Tc and Iodine 123 (^{123}I).

X rays emitted from atomic orbitals are sometimes used instead of gamma rays for imaging purposes. This is the case in cardiac imaging using the radionuclide thallium 201 (^{201}Tl). Usually, however, x rays from radionuclide studies are by-products that have no diagnostic value but do contribute to irradiation of the patient.

Electrons emitted from atomic orbitals as a result of nuclear radioactivi-

---

*There is one exception. Photons used in positron emission tomography result from positron decay of a nucleus. The photons are created outside the nucleus. However, they are often called gamma rays because of their high energy (511 keV). This is discussed in more detail later in this section.

ty originating from within the same atom usually travel less than 1 mm in tissue and contribute only to biologic effects. They provide no diagnostic information. Most radionuclides used in medical imaging have associated atomic orbital emissions. For example, although ^{99m}Tc and ^{123}I emit no beta particles from their nucleus, they do emit orbital electrons.

As mentioned earlier, in diagnostic radiography, x rays are electronically produced with a switch and are present only for a brief moment. Radionuclides, on the other hand, are created in nuclear reactors or at institutions having particle accelerators called *cyclotrons*. The radionuclides are shipped to the hospital either in ready-to-use form or in kits from which the proper radiopharmaceuticals can later be prepared. The radioactivity of an agent will be present for a long time compared to the brief existence of radiographic x rays.

To understand this, it must be realized that even a small sample of a radioactive agent is made up of billions of atoms, each of which can spontaneously emit the gamma rays, beta particles, electrons, and x rays specific to it. When a radioactive atom starts emitting the radiations, it emits all of them at once. After this, that atom no longer emits radiation and is "dead." When any one "live" nucleus will emit radiation cannot be predicted. However, it is possible to predict the percent of "live" nuclei that will emit their radiation within a given period of time. The time it takes for half the nuclei to emit their radiation is called the *physical half-life*. For example, for ^{99m}Tc nuclei, half emit their radiation within 6 hours. Of those nuclei remaining, half will emit their radiation in the next 6 hours. The radioactivity decreases by a factor of 2 every 6 hours until all nuclei are "dead." For ^{99m}Tc, the physical half-life is 6 hours. At 2 days, less than 0.005 of the original nuclei are still "alive." Appendix C lists physical half-lives for radionuclides commonly used in nuclear radiology.

The amount of time that radioactivity remains within a patient depends on the rate at which the patient eliminates the agent from her system by excretion as well as on the physical half-life of the radionuclide. In some cases, the agent may be rapidly eliminated through the urinary tract and remain in the patient only a very short time, even though the physical half-life of the radionuclide may be relatively long. The amount of time that it takes the patient to eliminate half of the radioactive agent by excretory means is referred to as the *biological half-life*. The biologic and the physical half-lives combine to determine how long radioactivity remains within a patient.

Concentration of a radiopharmaceutical in an organ of the body confines biologic effects primarily to that organ. Since beta radiations travel only about 1 mm in tissue, all their resultant ionization is confined to the organ in which they reside. However, because gamma rays can penetrate a significant amount of tissue, they can cause ionization in other organs a dis-

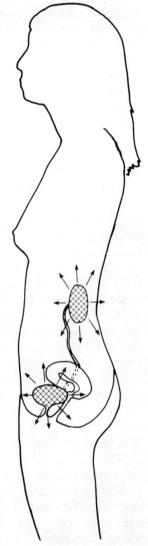

DTPA labeled
with Tc-99m
is filtered by kidneys
and excreted through
urinary tract. Gamma
rays from bladder are
the primary contributers
to conceptus irradiation.

FIG. 1-5. Irradiation of the conceptus from radionuclides in the maternal organs.

tance away. For pregnant patients, radiation reaches the embryo or fetus in two ways. The first is from the penetrating gamma rays and x rays of radiopharmaceuticals concentrated in maternal organs or in the placenta. The second is from radionuclides taken up by the organs of the embryo or fetus after they cross the placenta. The latter is sometimes more important, because the conceptus is irradiated not only by the x rays and gamma rays but additionally by any beta or orbital electron radiation that may be present.

Figure 1-5 shows the situation in which a mother receives the radiopharmaceutical diethylenetriamine pentaacetic acid (DTPA) labeled with ^{99m}Tc. Normally, this radiopharmaceutical is rapidly excreted by the urinary tract. The primary source of radiation to the fetus arises from the concentration of the radionuclide within the maternal urinary bladder. Additional contributions arise from concentrations generally distributed throughout the blood pool and from concentrations in the kidneys. The contribution of radiation from radionuclides within the placenta and the organs of the embryo or fetus is unknown because placental transfer is not well-documented for this labeled compound. It is assumed to be small compared to the radiation received from the mother's bladder.

On the other hand, Figure 1-6 demonstrates the case in which a mother receives a radioiodine thyroid scan. Irradiation of the conceptus from gamma rays originating from the thyroid of the mother is very small because of the distance of her thyroid from the conceptus. Radionuclides in the urine contribute more to conceptus irradiation.

Irradiation of the fetal thyroid depends in a large degree on the amount of radioactivity crossing the placenta and the percent of uptake by the fetal thyroid. This depends on conception age, and it is known that uptake can be large if the radioiodine is administered after the thyroid begins functioning at around 8 weeks postconception (Dyer and Brill, 1969). It should be remembered that the radioiodine, once taken up by the thyroid, remains there for a long time, and elimination is primarily dependent on the physical half-life of the isotope.

^{131}I is the most readily available and inexpensive radioisotope of iodine. The physical half-life of ^{131}I is 8.1 days, and the radioactivity decreases gradually over a period of many weeks. In addition, ^{131}I emits beta radiation that increases the amount of ionization in the organ. ^{123}I is less available and more expensive. However, it emits no beta particles from the nucleus and only a limited amount of low-energy atomic electrons. Additionally, its physical half-life is only 13 hours. Tissue ionization by ^{123}I will be far less than that by ^{131}I and is preferred for diagnostic studies.

INJURY FROM IONIZING RADIATION

Cell damage

The previous discussions have provided background in order to understand the mechanisms for biologic damage from ionizing radiations. Radiation may directly ionize a vital molecule in a cell. This is referred to as *direct* action. In *indirect* action, a molecule such as water may be ionized or excited. This water molecule may break up and produce highly reactive

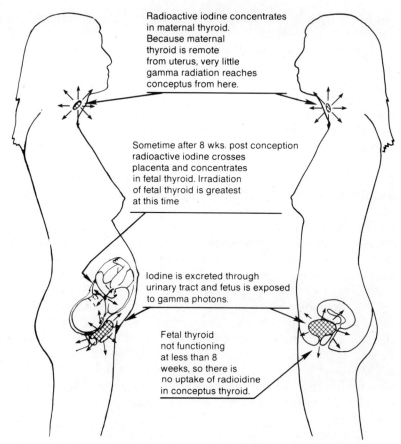

Radioactive iodine concentrates in maternal thyroid. Because maternal thyroid is remote from uterus, very little gamma radiation reaches conceptus from here.

Sometime after 8 wks. post conception radioactive iodine crosses placenta and concentrates in fetal thyroid. Irradiation of fetal thyroid is greatest at this time

Iodine is excreted through urinary tract and fetus is exposed to gamma photons.

Fetal thyroid not functioning at less than 8 weeks, so there is no uptake of radioidine in conceptus thyroid.

FIG. 1-6.   Radiation exposure to the fetus from free radioiodine.

chemical components called *free radicals* (single atoms or molecules having an unpaired electron). Chemical interactions can ensue and injure a vital molecule.

Damage to the genetic code is a well-known effect of ionizing radiations. (See, for instance, Pizzarello and Witcofski, 1982; Hall, 1978; and Travis, 1975.) The sensitivity of chromosomes to radiation is extensively documented. The arms of chromosomes may break up, or the centromere may be damaged. This injury may be repaired, or the genetic code may be rearranged or altered. The phenomenon may result in no observable change in cell function, some immediate dysfunction, or cell death. If the cell divides, the genetic alteration may be so severe as to be fatal upon replication. More significantly, the cell may remain viable and pass the defect on to daughter cells. Another possibility is that chromosomal damage may cause complications in cell replication, resulting in daughter cells with a deficiency or surplus of genetic information. Which of these effects, if any, that will take place as a result of ionization cannot be predicted because such events occur randomly.

Damage to the conceptus

The somatic consequence of cellular effects for conceptuses and their progeny is a more complex phenomenon that is not very well understood at present. Following are some possible effects:

- If only a few cells are involved, immunologic mechanisms may recognize the aberrant ones, destroy them, and replace them with healthy cells.
- If the cells are not replaced, growth impairment of organs may result without functional damage. The child may be smaller than usual, but otherwise normal.
- On the other hand, damage to the cells may interrupt some crucial stage of development from which recovery is not possible, resulting in a deformity.
- Other somatic defects may also occur but may be too subtle to be noticed.
- It is possible that the damage may result in a neoplasm, which will remain unexpressed for many years.
- Gonadal damage may result that could, theoretically, affect the conceptus' progeny but not the conceptus itself.

The sensitivity of a conceptus to radiation depends on the degree of mitotic activity of the cells, the magnitude of and the delivery rate of the radiation, and the maturity of the developing offspring.

Mitotic activity. Bergonié and Tribondeau (1906) have shown that highly mitotic cells are most susceptible to permanent damage. This is sometimes referred to as the *Law of Bergonié and Tribondeau.* This "law" is not always valid, and major exceptions exist. Generally speaking, considerably more radiation is required to destroy the functional capacity of nonproliferating cells (*e.g.,* mature muscle) than to destroy the replicative capacity of proliferating ones (*e.g.,* stem cells). For this reason, the developing conceptus is thought to be more sensitive to radiation than is the mature adult, and its sensitivity to radiation may be greater during periods when cell division is more rapid.

Magnitude of damage. Somatic expression of cellular effects in a conceptus depends on the number of cells initially injured. Correspondingly, the number of injured cells depends on the amount of radiation delivered. If many cells are injured, the developing child is faced with a more complex problem than with single-cell injury. For repair to be complete, it must either repair the injured cells or destroy them and replace them with healthy ones. The task becomes increasingly more difficult as the number of injured cells increases. For large-scale injury, the repair may be incomplete, and permanent cell depletion may occur, leading to growth impairment, deformities, or death.

Rate of injury.   The success of cellular repair in a developing conceptus is dependent not only on the extent of injury to the organism, but also on the rate at which the cellular injury occurs. If injury occurs continually but at low levels, recovery mechanisms may be able to handle the load without serious organ injury or permanent cell depletion. The organism may continue to grow while repairing or replacing the injured cells. On the other hand, if the cumulative injury is delivered acutely, it might overburden the organism's corrective powers and result in permanent damage or death.

Maturity of the developing offspring.   Russell and Russell (1954) and Brent and Gorson (1972) demonstrated a correlation between conception age and radiation-induced malformations in mice and rats (Figs. 1-7 and 1-8). These experiments were carried out at dose levels considerably higher than those used in diagnostic radiology. They were designed to induce effects so that they could be correlated with gestation time. Resorption usually resulted when radiation was delivered prior to implantation. Prenatal death in the rodents could be induced by the radiation received during organogenesis but with an ever-decreasing incidence as it progressed. The crit-

FIG. 1-7.   Incidence of death and of abnormalities at term following irradiation with 200 R at various stages in the prenatal development of mice. The lower scale correlates conception age for humans. (Russell LB, Russell WL: An analysis of the changing radiation response of the developing mouse embryo. J Cell Physiol [Suppl 1]43:103, 1954)

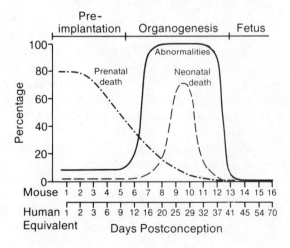

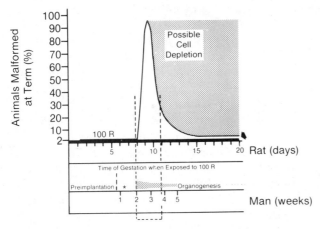

FIG. 1-8. Relative incidence of congenital malformations in the rat following an x-ray exposure of 100 R, delivered at various stages during gestation. The control incidence in this species is about 2%, indicated by the *arrow* on the right. The asterisk shows the stage of implantation when radiation causes growth retardation that is expressed as a decrease in weight at term. (Reproduced with permission from Brent RL, Gorson RO: Radiation exposure in pregnancy. In Moseley RD Jr et al (eds): Current Problems in Radiology. Copyright © 1972 by Year Book Medical Publishers, Inc., Chicago)

ical period for induced malformations occurred during this time. Malformation was much reduced when the radiation was delivered during the fetal stage (after organogenesis). Rugh (1964) demonstrated that specific radiation-induced malformations are correlated with the period of prenatal development critical to the malformed organism.

Although these data are useful, care must be exercised when extrapolating from animal data to potential consequences in the human. For example, the critical period of organ development in the rat or mouse is concurrent with major organogenesis. Dobbing and Sands (1973) have shown that the cerebral hemispheres in the human undergo rapid neuronal development during the 8th through 16th weeks postconception, while major organogenesis occurs before the 8th week. The timing of radiation exposure and radiation-induced cerebral anomalies in humans is not directly correlated to effects seen in rodents.

Dekaban (1968) studied 26 human conceptuses exposed to therapeutic levels of radiation (> 250 rad). From these data he made the following generalizations: (1) these large radiation doses delivered prior to 2 to 3 weeks postconception are not likely to result in severe abnormalities if the pregnancy continues; (2) if given between 4 and 11 weeks postconception, they lead to severe abnormalities of many organs in most or all of the exposed conceptuses; (3) similar doses delivered between 11 and 16 weeks postconception may result in stunted growth, microcephaly, or mental retardation; (4) if administered between 16 and 20 weeks postconception, they may lead to mild degrees of microcephaly, mental retardation, or stunted growth; and (5) after the 20th week postconception, these doses are not likely to produce debilitating abnormalities in early life.

These data are consistent with the general conclusion that organogenesis is the most susceptible stage for radiation-induced abnormalities, and that, prior to and after these stages, major abnormalities are not likely to result. However, it must be remembered that even though the period of major organogenesis in the human extends from the second through about the seventh week postconception, developmental organization of the brain does not take place until later stages.

There are teratogenic factors associated with some radionuclide studies that are not associated with externally delivered radiation. Stoffer and Hamburger (1976) have investigated the consequences of thyroid ablation treatment using ^{131}I on pregnant patients. They noted that the incidence of neonatal hypothyroidism increased if the treatment was administered beyond the eighth week postconception. This correlation is consistent with the onset of fetal thyroid function and points out the risks from placental transfer of radionuclides.

Nonionizing Radiations

ULTRASOUND EXAMINATIONS

Ultrasound is a nonionizing radiation. Sound waves are mechanical compression waves whereby a medium, such as air or tissue, is alternately compressed or stretched over short distances (Fig. 1-9). This compressing and stretching sets up a longitudinal vibratory wave that propagates through matter. A single compression and stretch represents one vibration, and the rate at which the vibrations take place is the frequency. The distance between compressions is the wavelength.

Humans perceive an increase in sound frequency as an increase in pitch. However, if the frequency gets too high, it becomes inaudible. These high-frequency sound waves are referred to as *ultrasound*. Conventional sound is on the order of several thousand vibrations per second, but ultrasound used in diagnostic radiology is on the order of 1 to 10 million vibrations per second. In tissue, the wavelength of ultrasound is less than 1 mm.

As used in diagnostic applications, ultrasound is initiated by a transducer that starts the compressing and stretching of the tissue medium. The

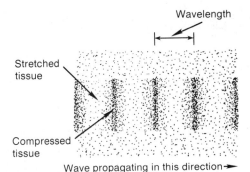

FIG. 1-9. Sound waves propagating through tissue.

transducer not only makes the sound, it also receives it. To create an image, a short burst or pulse of ultrasound of about a millionth of a second duration is delivered. The transducer then ceases its sound-producing activity and listens for about a thousandth of a second for reflections or echoes of the sound. Thus, only a few tenths of one percent of the time is spent producing sound; the rest is spent receiving it. This sequence is repeated about a thousand times every second.

Echoes are created at interfaces or boundaries of organs, tissues, fluids, or gases that have different acoustic properties. The speed of ultrasound in tissue is 0.154 cm per microsecond. The time interval between the transmission of the sound pulse and the reception of its echo is determined by the depth of the boundary in the body. Figure 1-10 demonstrates this pulse–echo principle. Ultrasound images are therefore maps of acoustic interfaces between biologic materials in the body. By applying the transducer at different angles, boundaries can be viewed from different directions to improve the field of view of the image. Since the uterus, placenta, amniotic fluid, fat, and so on have different acoustic properties, their boundaries can be mapped by ultrasound to form a two-dimensional image.

Some ultrasound systems do not operate in the previously described pulse–echo mode. If two transducers are used so that one serves only to produce sound while the other is used only to listen to the echoes, the sound-producing transducer can continually send while the listening transducer receives. This technique is called the *continuous-wave mode.*

Ultrasound may be used to monitor fetal heartbeat in a nonimaging mode. Moving objects also cause echoes. However, the motion of the object changes the incident sound into an echo of a different frequency. The echoed frequency depends on the velocity of the moving object. This phenomenon, known as the Doppler effect, permits the ultrasonographer to monitor quantitatively the movement of the fetal mitral valve and the flow of blood.

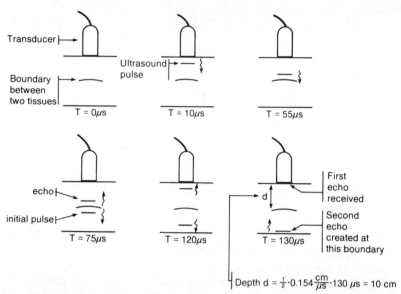

FIG. 1-10. Pulse-echo principle of ultrasound imaging. Time is expressed in microseconds (μs) or millionths of a second.

Although Figures 1-9 and 1-10 demonstrate the principles of echo production and image formation, they do not accurately demonstrate sound-wave propagation in tissues. The intensity of each pulse is not the same at all points along its path of propagation. Transverse to its path, the sound intensity is maximal in the center and tapers off to zero at the edges. Furthermore, the central intensity of each pulse varies along the path of propagation. It initially increases because of focusing as the sound wave moves away from the transducer, reaches a maximum at some distance from the transducer, and then spreads out and continually decreases beyond the maximum. The actual depth where the sound is most intense depends on the physical design of the transducer, the composition of the tissues, and the frequency of the ultrasound.

Another important point is that the transducer is moved during a scan to sweep the field of view. A conceptus is often outside the path of the sound pulses, and thus the amount of time that it is actually exposed to the sound is limited.

MECHANISMS FOR EFFECTS FROM ULTRASOUND

The rapid compressing and stretching of tissues by sound waves may lead to biologic injury from ultrasound. The extent to which sound waves affect tissues is dependent on the frequency, intensity, duration, and mode of application of the sound as well as on the composition of the tissues. A comprehensive review is available in NCRP (1983).

As an ultrasound wave passes through tissues, its mechanical energy is converted to other forms (Wells, 1977; Hussey, 1975; Nyborg, 1977; Hill, 1977; Kremkau, 1983; NCRP, 1983). The mechanisms for this conversion are not completely understood but may result in a rise in tissue temperature. This effect is sometimes used in cancer therapy to destroy tumors. The maximal attainable temperature depends on how quickly the heat is conducted away from the organism and how effectively the body's temperature-controlling mechanisms respond. It also depends on the rate at which the energy is delivered and the method of application (sweeping or nonsweeping beam, pulse–echo or continuous mode). The energy delivered to tissues from therapeutic ultrasonic procedures is considerably greater than that delivered by diagnostic ultrasound, and extrapolation of effects from one to the other is not possible. However, diagnostic ultrasound may not be completely harmless, and heat generation is one mechanism for possible biologic effects.

Sound-wave energy may also "jostle" micron-sized gas bubbles within tissues. This is referred to as *cavitation*. In order for cavitation to exist, micron-sized bubbles must already be present in tissues. The vibratory motion of a bubble attracts diffused gases to feed and enlarge it. Under extreme conditions, a pulsating bubble can be forced to collapse. This collapse can lead to the production of free radicals within the gas filling the bubble. These may subsequently diffuse into the tissues and cause biologic effects. The process is slow and is not likely to occur at diagnostic levels because there is too much time between pulses to sustain the phenomenon. Cavitation is more significant in therapeutic applications of ultrasound.

Pulsating bubbles can also resemble more of a distorted pulsation than a spherically symmetrical one. Distorted pulsations give rise to a stirring of the fluids near the surface of the bubble. This stirring causes eddylike currents called *microstreams* that result in rapid rotation and reorientation of macromolecules (*e.g.*, DNA). In addition, fluid velocities created by this stirring can be very different over short distances. Macromolecules caught in different velocity currents can be sheared by the forces they create.

Areas where fluid velocities change rapidly over short distances can also be created by the vibratory motion of other inhomogeneities within tissues. The "churning" of tissue fluids near such inhomogeneities may again result in disruption of molecules or membranes near these velocity gradients.

Most of these mechanisms have been demonstrated in fluids, but their presence in humans at diagnostic levels has not been confirmed. It is not known if the physical composition of tissues (*e.g.*, are microbubbles present?) and the manner of ultrasound delivery (*e.g.*, pulsed vs. continuous) are conducive to such effects.

Many researchers have reported on observations of biologic effects induced by diagnostic levels of ultrasound. Some effects have been produced in amphibian embryos and insect larvae suspended in fluids (Sarvazyan et al, 1982; Pizzarello et al, 1978; Child et al, 1981). The data are sometimes contradictory. Pizzarello and co-workers (1978) observed the presence of miniature flies developing from sonicated larvae. Under similar conditions, Child and associates (1980) were unable to reproduce this effect.

Several investigators have observed ultrasonically induced effects on cells cultured *in vitro* (Siegel et al, 1979; Liebeskind et al, 1979a, 1979b, 1981, 1982; Miller et al, 1979; Pinamonti et al 1982). Liebeskind and associates (1979a, 1981) have observed morphological changes in cultured cells and have demonstrated effects that suggest damage to DNA.

The effect receiving the most attention is sister chromatid exchange because this is a sensitive indicator for possible mutagenic and carcinogenic agents. Jacobson-Kram (1984) has reviewed 12 articles on the subject (Au et al, 1982; Barnett et al, 1982; Barrass et al, 1982; Haupt et al, 1981; Liebeskind et al, 1979a, 1979b; Lundberg et al, 1982; Miller et al, 1983; Morris et al, 1978; Wegner et al, 1980, 1982; Zheng et al, 1981). Nine reported on sonication of cells cultured *in vitro*. Seven of these found no effect, while two studies were positive. The causes of the discrepancies are uncertain. Two studies were done on human amniotic fluid sonicated *in vivo*. No significant effect was found in either case. One study investigated sister chromatid exchange on conceptuses of pregnant mice. No significant effect was found.

In vivo animal investigations have been performed (Anderson and Barrett, 1981; Kremkau and Witcofski, 1974; Miller et al, 1976). Kremkau and Witcofski (1974) reported mitotic reduction in rat liver exposed to ultrasound. However, Miller and co-workers (1976) were unable to reproduce these results in similar experiments. The reasons for this discrepancy are unknown.

These studies are necessary in order to understand what effects might be anticipated, how the effects might be caused, and what the results might be. Because the bioeffects of diagnostic ultrasound critically depend on the environment of exposed tissues and on the manner of delivery of ultrasound, it is not possible to make valid extrapolations from these observations to the possible consequences diagnostic ultrasound might have on a human conceptus.

MAGNETIC RESONANCE EXAMINATIONS

Magnetic resonance (MR) is a relatively recent development that is noninvasive, uses no ionizing radiations, and employs the interaction of four magnetic fields in order to acquire an image. These fields are

1. The magnetic field (or magnetic moment) of atomic nuclei (usually hydrogen proton nuclei) that naturally exist in the human body
2. A strong, static, uniform magnetic field in which a patient lies
3. A weaker magnetic-field gradient added to the uniform field in order to encode spatial information into the data
4. A magnetic field associated with radiofrequency (RF) waves, the same kind as those used by FM broadcasting stations

When a patient lies in a strong, externally applied magnetic field (Fig. 1-11), the magnetic atomic nuclei in her body align themselves parallel or antiparallel to it. Most align themselves in a parallel fashion. This preferential alignment can be reversed by application of pulsed RF waves of a specific (one and only one) frequency. The required frequency depends on the magnetic moment of the nuclei being imaged and the strength of the magnetic field in which they reside. If all hydrogen proton nuclei reside in the same externally applied magnetic field, they all respond at the same frequency. However, if the strength of the externally applied field varies at different points inside the patient, the response frequency of hydrogen proton nuclei depends on where they are located. This phenomenon can be used to decipher spatial information when constructing the image. Variations in the magnetic-field strength at different positions in the body are achieved through externally applied, weak magnetic-field gradients (Fig. 1-11, *c*).

FIG. 1-11. Magnetic resonance (MR).

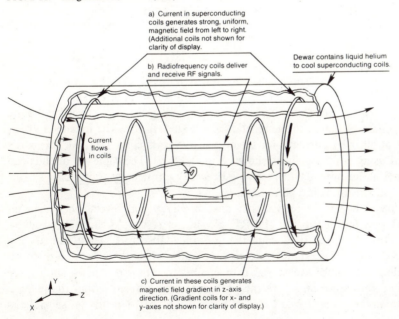

a) Current in superconducting coils generates strong, uniform, magnetic field from left to right. (Additional coils not shown for clarity of display.

b) Radiofrequency coils deliver and receive RF signals.

Dewar contains liquid helium to cool superconducting coils.

Current flows in coils

c) Current in these coils generates magnetic field gradient in z-axis direction. (Gradient coils for x- and y-axes not shown for clarity of display.)

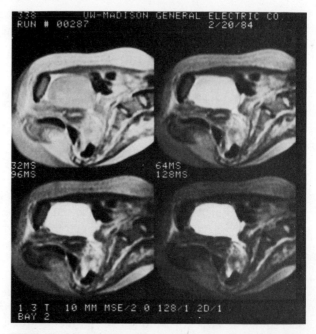

FIG. 1-12. Magnetic resonance sagittal images of a female pelvis in a supine position. Each image was acquired using slightly different data-acquisition sequences. Note in this case that the nongravida uterus is behind the relatively full bladder and is located at central depth in the pelvis. This is a *retroverted* uterus as confirmed by laparoscopy. (Reproduced with permission from the General Electric Co.)

The strong, external, uniform magnetic field can be applied using superconducting, resistive, or permanent magnets. Figure 1-11 shows the use of a superconducting magnet. Electric current in the superconducting coils generates the strong magnetic field (Fig. 1-11, *a*). The magnetic gradient is applied by current in a set of resistive coils (Fig. 1-11, *c*). RF is delivered using copper coils as shown (Fig. 1-11, *b*). The same set of coils can be used as an antenna to receive RF energy emitted by the nuclei, as discussed in the following paragraph.

When RF acts on nuclei, they absorb energy and reverse their orientation. Upon termination of the RF, the nuclei return to their initial alignment. In doing so, they emit the RF they absorbed. These signals are detected and, after some data manipulation, their frequency and corresponding intensities are stored in a computer. The frequencies supply the spatial information on where the signals originated from within the patient. The intensity of each frequency is information that depends on several tissue properties, including the number of hydrogen proton nuclei present, their fluid motion, if any, and the time it takes for the nuclei to reorient themselves after an RF pulse. The latter is called *relaxation time* and has two components, T1 and T2, each of which depends on the biochemical environment of the nuclei within the patient.

The reconstructed image therefore represents some combination of the proton density, the two relaxation times, and the flow, if any. Different RF pulse sequences can be used to place emphasis on one or more of these parameters. This results in images that look different and have different diagnostic value (Fig. 1-12).

An MR image is displayed on a console (Fig. 1-12), and it looks similar to that of a CT image; however, the information is considerably different. This is because MR images are related to the biochemical environment of nuclei, while CT images represent the x-ray attenuation properties of tissues in the patient.

In a routine examination, once the patient is positioned within the magnet, the desired pulse-imaging sequence is initiated. Typically, an RF pulse of a few microseconds' duration is delivered. Following the RF pulse, the computer controls the electric currents in the gradient coils in order to encode spatial information, and the receiver detects the signals from the nuclei. This sequence is repeated many times during the examination, which will usually last about an hour.

MECHANISMS FOR EFFECTS FROM MR

Budinger (1981), Saunders (1982), Mansfield and Morris (1982), and Saunders and Orr (1983) have reviewed the mechanisms and known effects from RF radiation and magnetic fields typically used in MR. In considering possible mechanisms for biologic effects, we consider separately those effects from

1. Strong, externally applied, static magnetic fields
2. Rapidly changing magnetic-field gradients
3. RF waves

Some mechanisms are hypothesized from the known laws of physics and have as yet to be demonstrated in biologic systems; others have produced observable responses in animals. These latter observed responses have been benign and inconsequential to the animal's health except for situations far in excess of those encountered in medical imaging. Although no immediate biologic consequences of MR are anticipated, possible long-term effects cannot be ruled out. No detailed long-term epidemiologic studies have investigated such effects. It should be noted that, as currently used, all studies investigating possible mutagenic effects have been negative.

An electrostatic potential difference can be generated across a conducting fluid (*i.e.,* blood) moving through a static magnetic field. The presence of such potentials generated across the great vessels and hearts of animals have been observed in electrocardiograms (ECGs) (Beischer and Knepton, 1964; Beischer, 1969; Togawa et al, 1967; Gaffey et al 1980). The observed potentials are on the order of millivolts and have no apparent adverse effects at magnetic-field strengths currently used in MR imaging (less than 2 tesla*). Saunders (1982) reports observing no changes in the ECGs of humans during or after imaging.

Forces are exerted on charged particles that move through magnetic fields. This phenomenon has been proposed to explain observed effects on the electric impulses of nerves resting in strong static magnetic fields (Reno, 1969; Kolta, 1973). However, contradictory evidence suggests that these observations are artifacts of experimental conditions. No significant effects have been demonstrated by recent research using static magnetic fields similar to those employed in medical imaging (Schwartz, 1978; Gaffey and Tenoforde, 1980).

There have been other suggestions of possible cellular damage and occupationally related skin effects from exposure to static magnetic fields (Malinin et al, 1976; Vyalov, 1974). However, subsequent experiments and experiences of other groups are contradictory and strongly suggest that observed effects are due to causes other than magnetic fields (Frazier, 1980; also see Budinger, 1981). The scientific evidence for possible deleterious effects from static magnetic fields used in MR is not compelling. At this time, experience indicates no deleterious effects from static magnetic fields of less than 2 tesla.

Electric currents can be induced in objects that reside in changing magnetic fields. In order to develop spatial information, the magnetic-field gradients are switched on and off in sequence with the RF pulses. These changing magnetic-field gradients can induce currents in the patient. Any possible deleterious effects from induction of such currents depend on the magnitude and the time dependence of the changing magnetic field. As used in MR, the induced currents are so small that no deleterious effects are anticipated.

Changing magnetic fields have been shown to induce visual light flashes called *phosphenes* (d'Arsonval, 1896; Barlow et al, 1947; Lövsund et al, 1980). There is a threshold, dependent on magnetic-field intensity and the frequency of the changing field, below which this phenomenon is not apparent. No reports of phosphenes have been published for MR devices.

Heat generation is the primary mechanism for potential biologic effects from RF radiation. Heating depends strongly on the frequency of the radia-

---

*A tesla is a unit of magnetic field strength. See Chapter 2.

tion, the manner of exposure to the radiation, and the intensity. In diagnostic imaging, deleterious effects from heating are not anticipated and have not been experienced.

Much attention is given to possible mutagenic effects of radiations used in diagnostic imaging because of the implication such effects may have for carcinogenesis. Several studies on these effects have recently appeared in the literature (Geard et al, 1984; Wolff et al, 1980; Schwartz and Crooks, 1982; Thomas and Morris, 1981; Cooke and Morris, 1981). No observable mutations, sister chromatid exchange, or other effects have been reported from MR as used in medical imaging.

Other mechanisms exist, but the consequences seem negligible (Budinger, 1981; Mansfield and Morris, 1982). At this time, the known mechanisms and effects appear to be inconsequential. Further investigation of possible mechanisms for effects is needed because of the potential for widespread application of MR imaging in pregnant women.

References

Anderson DW, Barrett JT: Depression of phagocytosis by ultrasound. Ultrasound Med Biol 7:267, 1981

Au WW, Obergoenner N, Goldenthal KL et al: Sister chromatid exchanges in mouse embryos after exposure to ultrasound *in utero*. Mutat Res 103:315, 1982

Barlow HB, Kohn HI, Walsh EG: Visual sensations aroused by magnetic fields. Am J Physiol 148:372, 1947

Barnett SB, Bonin A, Mitchell G et al: An investigation of the mutagenic potential of pulsed ultrasound. Br J Radiol 55:501, 1982

Barrass N, Ter Haar G, Casey G: The effect of ultrasound and hyperthermia on sister chromatid exchange and division kinetics of BHK21 C13/A3 cells. Br J Cancer (Suppl V) 4:187, 1982

Beischer DE: Vectorcardiogram and aortic blood flow of squirrel monkeys (*Saimiri sciureus*) in a strong superconductive electromagnet. In Barnothy MF (ed): Biological Effects of Magnetic Fields, Vol 2, pp 241–259. New York, Plenum Press, 1969

Beischer DE, Knepton JC: Influence of strong magnetic fields on the electrocardiogram of squirrel monkeys (*Saimiri sciureus*). Aerospace Med 35:939, 1964

Bergonié J, Tribondeau L: De quelques résultats de la radiothérapie et essai de fixation d'une technique rationelle. Comptes Rendus Acad Sci (Paris) 143:983, 1906

Brent RL, Gorson RO: Radiation exposure in pregnancy. Curr Probl Radiology 2:1, 1972

Budinger TF: Nuclear magnetic resonance (NMR) *in vivo* studies: Known thresholds for health effects. J Comput Assist Tomogr 5:800, 1981

Child SZ, Carstensen EL, Davis HT: Test for "miniature flies" following exposure of drosophilia melanogaster larvae to diagnostic levels of ultrasound. Exp Cell Biol 48:461, 1980

Child SZ, Carstensen EL, Lam SK: Effects of ultrasound on Drosophila: III. Exposure of larvae to low-temporal average-intensity, pulsed irradiation. Ultrasound Med Biol 7:167, 1981

Cooke P, Morris PG: The effects of NMR exposure on living organisms. II. A genetic study of human lymphocytes. Br J Radiol 54:622, 1981

d'Arsonval MA: Dispositifs pour la mesure des courants alternatifs a toutes frequences. Comptes Rendus des Seances. Societe de Biologie et de Filiales et Associees (Paris) 3:451, 1896

Dekaban AS: Abnormalities in children exposed to x-radiation during various stages of gestation: Tentative timetable of radiation injury to the human fetus. Part I. J Nucl Med 9:471, 1968

Dobbing J, Sands J: Quantitative growth and development of human brain. Arch Dis Child 48:757, 1973

Dyer NC, Drill B: Fetal radiation dose from maternally administered ^{59}Fe and ^{131}I. In Sikov MR, Mahlum DD (eds): Radiation Biology of the Fetal and Juvenile Mammal, pp 73–88. Oak Ridge, Tennessee, USAEC, Division of Technical Information, 1969

Frazier ME: Biological effects of magnetic fields: A progress report. In Rem WN, Archer VE (eds): Health Implications of New Energy Technologies, pp 679–685. Ann Arbor, Michigan, Ann Arbor Science Publishers, 1980

Gaffey CT, Tenforde TS: Electrical properties of conducting frog sciatic nerves exposed to high DC magnetic fields. Bioelectromagnetics 1:208, 1980

Gaffey CT, Tenforde TS, Dean EE: Alterations in the electrocardiograms of baboons exposed to DC magnetic fields. Bioelectromagnetics 1:209, 1980

Geard CR, Osmak RS, Hall EJ et al: Magnetic resonance and ionizing radiation: A comparative evaluation *in-vitro* of oncogenic and genotoxic potential. Radiology 152:199, 1984

Hall EJ: Radiobiology for the Radiologist, 2nd ed, pp 51–61, 385–395. New York, Harper and Row, 1978

Haupt M, Martin AO, Simpson JL et al: Ultrasound induction of sister chromatid exchanges in human lymphocytes. Hum Genet 59:221, 1981

Hill CR: Biological effects of ultrasound. In Wells PNT (ed): Ultrasonics in Clinical Diagnosis, pp 171–180. New York, Churchill-Livingstone, 1977

Hussey M: Diagnostic Ultrasound, pp 12–45. London, Blackie and Son, 1975

Jacobson-Kram D: The effects of diagnostic ultrasound on sister chromatid exchange frequencies: A review of the recent literature. J Clin Ultrasound 12:5, 1984

Kolta P: Strong and permanent interaction between peripheral nerve and a constant inhomogeneous magnetic field. Acta Physiol Acad Sci Hung 43:89, 1973

Kremkau FW: Biological effects and possible hazards. Clin Obstet Gynaecol 10:395, 1983

Kremkau FW, Witcofski RL: Mitotic reduction in rat liver exposed to ultrasound. J Clin Ultrasound 2:123, 1974

Liebeskind D, Bases R, Elequin F et al: Diagnostic ultrasound: Effects on the DNA and growth patterns of animal cells. Radiology 131:177, 1979a

Liebeskind D, Bases R, Koenigsberg M et al: Morphological changes in the surface characteristics of cultured cells after exposure to diagnostic ultrasound. Radiology 138:419, 1981

Liebeskind D, Bases R, Mendez F et al: Sister chromatid exchanges in human lymphocytes after exposure to diagnostic ultrasound. Science 205:1273, 1979b

Liebeskind D, Padawer J, Wolley R et al: Diagnostic ultrasound: Time-lapse and transmission electron microscopic studies of cells isonated *in vitro*. Br J Cancer (Suppl V) 45:176, 1982

Lövsund P, Nilsson SEG, Reuter T et al: Magneto phosphenes: A quantitative analysis of thresholds. Med Biol Eng Comput 18:326, 1980

Lundberg M, Jerominski L, Livingston G et al: Failure to demonstrate an effect of *in vivo* diagnostic ultrasound on sister chromatid exchange frequency in amniotic fluid cells. Am J Med Genet 11:31, 1982

Malinin GI, Gregory WD, Morelli L et al: Evidence of morphological and physiological transformation of mammalian cells by strong magnetic fields. Science 194:844, 1976

Mansfield P, Morris PG: NMR Imaging in Biomedicine, pp 297–332. New York, Academic Press, 1982

Miller DL, Nyborg WL, Whitcomb CC: Platelet aggregation induced by ultrasound under specialized conditions *in vitro*. Science 205:505, 1979

Miller MW, Kaufman GE, Cataldo FL et al: Absence of mitotic reduction in regenerating rat livers exposed to ultrasound. J Clin Ultrasound 4:169, 1976

Miller MW, Wolff S, Filly R et al: Absence of an effect of diagnostic ultrasound on sister-chromatid exchange induction in human lymphocytes *in vitro*. Mutat Res 120:261, 1983

Morris SM, Palmer CG, Fry FJ et al: Effect of ultrasound on human leucocytes. Sister chromatid exchange analysis. Ultrasound Med Biol 4:253, 1978

NCRP (National Council on Radiation Protection and Measurements): Biological Effects of Ultrasound: Mechanisms and Clinical Implications, Report No. 74. Bethesda, Maryland, National Council on Radiation Protection and Measurements, 1983

Nyborg WL: Physical Mechanisms for Biological Effects of Ultrasound, HEW publication (FDA) 78-8062. Rockville, Maryland, Bureau of Radiological Health, 1977

Pinamonti S, Gallenga PE, Mazzeo V: Effect of pulsed ultrasound on human erythrocytes *in vitro*. Ultrasound Med Biol 8:631, 1982

Pizzarello DJ, Vivino A, Madden B et al: Effect of pulsed low-power ultrasound on growing tissues. I. Developing mammalian and insect tissue. Exp Cell Biol 46:179, 1978

Pizzarello DJ, Witcofski RL: Medical Radiation Biology, 2nd ed pp 15–41. Philadelphia, Lea and Febiger, 1982

Reno VR: Conduction Velocity in Nerve Exposed to a High Magnetic Field, NASA Report No. NAMI-1089, Government Printing Office, Washington DC, 1969

Rugh R: Why Radiobiology? Radiology 82:917, 1964

Russell LB, Russell WL: An analysis of the changing radiation response of the developing mouse embryo. J Cell Physiol (Suppl 1) 43:103, 1954

Sarvazyan AP, Beloussov LV, Petropavlovskaya MN et al: The action of low-intensity pulsed ultrasound on amphibian embryonic tissues. Ultrasound Med Biol 8:639, 1982

Saunders RD: Biological hazards of NMR. In Witcofski RL, Karstaedt N, Partain CL (eds): NMR Imaging, p. 65. Winston-Salem, North Carolina, The Bowman Gray School of Medicine, 1982

Saunders RD, Orr JS: Biologic effects on NMR. In Partain CL, James AE, Rollo FD, Price RR (eds): Nuclear Magnetic Resonance (NMR) Imaging, pp 383–396. Philadelphia, WB Saunders, 1983

Schwartz JL: Influence of a constant magnetic field on nervous tissue: I. Nerve conduction velocity studies. IEEE Trans Biomed Eng BME-25:467, 1978

Schwartz JL, Crooks LE: NMR imaging produces no observable mutations or cytoxicity in mammalian cells. Am J Radiol 139:583, 1982

Siegel E, Goddard J, James AE et al: Cellular attachment as a sensitive indicator of the effects of diagnostic ultrasound exposure on cultured human cells. Radiology 133:175, 1979

Stoffer SS, Hamburger JI: Inadvertent ^{131}I therapy for hypothyroidism in the first trimester in pregnancy. J Nucl Med 17:146, 1976

Thomas A, Morris PG: The effects of NMR exposure on living organisms. I. A microbial assay. Br J Radiol 54:615, 1981

Togawa T, Okai O, Oshima M: Observation of blood flow EMF in externally applied strong magnetic fields by surface electrodes. Med Biol Eng 5:169, 1967

Travis EL: Primer of Medical Radiobiology, pp 23–46 Chicago, Year Book Medical Publishers, 1975

Vyalov AM: Clinico–hygienic and experimental data on the effects of magnetic fields under industrial conditions. In Kholodov YA (ed): Influence of Magnetic Fields on Biological Objects, Joint Publ. Res. Service Rpt. 63038 pp 163–174. Springfield, Virginia, National Technical Information Service, 1974

Wegner R-D, Meyenburg M: The effects of diagnostic ultrasonography on frequencies of sister chromatid exchanges in Chinese hamster cells and human lymphocytes. J Ultrasound Med 1:355, 1982

Wegner R-D, Obe G, Meyenburg M: Has diagnostic ultrasound mutagenic effects? Hum Genet 56:95, 1980

Wells PNT: Basic principles. In Wells PNT (ed): Ultrasonics in Clinical Diagnosis, pp 3–17. New York, Churchill-Livingstone, 1977

Wolff S, Crooks LE, Brown P et al: Tests for DNA and chromasomal damage induced by nuclear magnetic resonance imaging. Radiology 136:707, 1980

Zheng HZ, Mitter NS, Chudley AE: *In vivo* exposure to diagnostic ultrasound and *in vitro* assay of sister chromatid exchanges in cultured amniotic fluid cells. IRCS Med Sci 9:491, 1981

Chapter 2
The Units
and Measures
of Radiations

The extent of biologic damage to an unborn child depends primarily on the amount of energy deposited in the child's tissues. It may also be related to the manner of application of the radiation or to forces exerted on tissues during the imaging sequence. It is therefore important to understand the measures and units of radiation. For x rays and gamma rays, quantities measured include exposure, absorbed dose, and absorbed dose equivalent. For radioisotopes, the administered radioactivity is measured by the disintegration or decay rate. With diagnostic ultrasound the amount of energy delivered is quantified in terms of integrated average power per unit area. For magnetic resonance, the magnetic-field strength and absorbed radiofrequency (RF) power are important. The units used in this text are those most commonly used in the United States. The international system of units (SI) is reviewed in Table 2-1.

Exposure

X rays and gamma rays cause ionization as they pass through air. The number of ions created is dependent on the number and energy of x rays or gamma rays passing through it. *Exposure is the amount of ionic charge created per unit mass of air by x- or gamma radiation less than 3 MeV.* It is measured in units called roentgen (R). One roentgen of x rays or gamma rays produces over 2 billion ion pairs per cubic centimeter of exposed air at

35

Table 2-1.   Conversion to SI Units

SI Unit	=	Conversion Factor	×	Other Unit
Exposure in mC/kg (mC/kg = millicoulomb per kilogram)	=	0.258	×	Exposure in R (R = roentgen)
Absorbed dose in Gy (Gy = Gray)	=	0.01	×	Absorbed dose in rd (rd = rad)
Absorbed dose in cGy (cGy = centigray)	=	1.0	×	Absorbed dose in rd (rd = rad)
Absorbed dose in cGy (cGy = centigray)	=	0.001	×	Absorbed dose in mrd (mrd = millirad)
Absorbed dose equivalent in Sv (Sv = Sievert)	=	0.01	×	Absorbed dose equivalent in rem
Activity in MBq (MBq = megabecquerel)	=	37	×	Activity in mCi (mCi = millicurie)
Activity in kBq (kBq = kilobecquerel)	=	37	×	Activity in μCi (μCi = microcurie)
Magnetic field in T (T = tesla)	=	0.0001	×	Magnetic field in G (G = gauss)

standard temperature and pressure. A word of caution: the inexperienced observer may confuse roentgen and milliroentgen exposures. A milliroentgen (mR) is an amount of radiation 1000 times less than that producing 1 roentgen exposure. A 20-mR exposure to a pregnant woman is considerably different from a 20-R exposure.

Absorbed Dose

Although exposure is an adequate quantification of diagnostic x rays and gamma rays emitted from a source, a more relevant measurement for biologic damage is the energy deposited in tissue through the interaction of ionizing radiations. *Absorbed dose is the energy imparted to tissue per unit mass of tissue.* It is measured in units of rad. One rad is strictly defined as the deposition of 0.01 joules of energy per kilogram of tissue. Conveniently, an exposure of 1 roentgen will yield an absorbed dose of roughly 1 rad. The same quantitative relation exists between rad and millirad as between roentgen and milliroentgen.

Absorbed Dose Equivalent

The unit of absorbed dose provides us with information regarding the amount of energy deposited per unit mass of tissue. However, radiobiologists have shown that different types of ionizing radiation cause different amounts of tissue damage even though the same dose of each type of radiation is delivered. This is particularly true for therapeutic radiations like neutrons. *Absorbed dose equivalent is defined as the product of the dose times a quality factor that takes into account the degree of effect that various radiations have on human tissue.* The common unit of absorbed dose equivalent is the rem and is the product of the quality factor times the dose in rad. For example, the quality factor for fast neutrons is usually assigned a value of 10. Therefore, 1 rad of neutrons would be an absorbed dose equivalent of 10 rem.

The quality factor for gamma rays is 1 and, therefore, a 1-rad dose of gamma radiation is a dose equivalent of 1 rem. In fact, the quality factor for all diagnostic radiations is 1, and we can equate

$$1 \text{ rem } = 1 \text{ rad } \approx 1 \text{ roentgen} \quad \text{(For diagnostic radiations)}$$

Therefore, these units, when applied to diagnostic radiology, are synonymous estimators of relative biologic risks.

Radioactivity

In nuclear radiology, the radiation dose absorbed by a conceptus depends on the amount of radioactivity administered. *Radioactivity is the rate at which nuclei in a sample undergo spontaneous emission of radiation.* This rate of spontaneous emission of radiation is sometimes referred to as the number of *disintegrations* per unit time and is directly proportional to the number of radionuclei present in the sample. The unit of radioactivity is the curie. The common specification of activity administered to a patient for diagnostic purposes is the millicurie (mCi) or the microcurie (μCi). A millicurie of activity is equivalent to 37 million disintegrations per second, and a microcurie of activity is equivalent to 37 thousand disintegrations per second.

The correlation between absorbed dose and the amount of radioactivity administered to a patient differs for each radiopharmaceutical. This is due to differences in the half-lives of radionuclides, differences in their radiative emissions, and differences in the metabolism of various radiopharmaceuticals. For example, because iodine 131 is a beta-emitting radionuclide and because it has a half-life of 8 days, the absorbed dose to the thyroid from a given administered activity will be significantly greater than the absorbed dose from the same administered activity of ^{99m}Tc pertechnetate. This is because this latter nuclide emits no beta radiation, has a half-life of only 6 hours, and is less readily taken up by the thyroid.

Integrated Ultrasound Intensity

Sound intensity is the measure of the amount of sound-wave energy that transverses a unit area of a patient's tissue per given amount of time. It is measured in terms of power (energy passing the tissue per unit time) per unit area of tissue. Note that this differs from the concept of absorbed dose. This is *not* a measurement of the amount of energy absorbed by tissues, only the amount incident. The common unit of measurement is watts per square centimeter (W/cm^2). The maximum intensity produced in the cross section of the ultrasound beam at its focus is called the *spatial peak intensity.* This intensity is commonly specified as a characteristic of the ultrasound delivered. Another intensity that is often quoted is the *spatial average intensity.* This is the intensity averaged over an appropriate area, typically the area of the transducer. For a given device the spatial average intensity would necessarily be less than the spatial peak intensity.

As previously mentioned, pulsed ultrasound transducers spend only a few tenths of one percent of their time emitting sound. The remainder is spent receiving echoes. When specifying sound intensities for biologic effects, it is conventional to average the intensity over time and to quote it in mW/cm^2. For example, if the spatial peak intensity delivered to tissue reaches $100\ W/cm^2$ when the transducer is emitting sound, but the sound exists for only 0.1 percent of the time, then the temporally averaged power per unit area is 1000 times less than the instantaneous level. In this case, the temporally averaged power per unit area is $0.1\ W/cm^2$ or $100\ mW/cm^2$.

Ultrasound intensity characteristic of a given transducer can be specified in four different ways:

1. The *spatial peak temporal peak* (SPTP) intensity is the maximum instantaneous intensity delivered by a device and is usually quoted in W/cm^2.
2. The *spatial average temporal peak* (SATP) intensity is the intensity averaged over an appropriate area (typically the area of the transducer face) at the moment when the ultrasound intensity is at its maximum (this value may be a factor of 2 to 200 less than the SPTP intensity).
3. The *spatial peak temporal average* (SPTA) intensity is the time-averaged intensity at the point in the medium where the intensity is maximum. (For pulsed imagers this is typically 300 to 1000 times less than the

SPTP intensity and ranges from 0.1 mW/cm^2 to 200 mW/cm^2 for commercial devices used in obstetrics.)
4. The *spatial average temporal average* (SATA) intensity is the intensity averaged over an appropriate area and also averaged over time. (This is typically thousands of times less than the SPTP intensity and is usually quoted in mW/cm^2.)

For consistency, we will adopt the *spatial peak temporal average* (SPTA) as the indicator of sound intensity. However, the reader should be aware of the different methods of quoting intensities when reading the literature.

Bioeffects that may result from ultrasound depend on the length of time during which the ultrasound is delivered. Integrated intensity takes into account the duration of the study and may be adequately summarized by quoting the intensity and the length of time that it is applied.

Magnetic-Field Strength

The SI units for magnetic-field strength is the tesla (T). The earth's magnetic field is on the order of 0.00005 T. Magnetic fields currently used for diagnostic imaging range from 0.03 T to 1.5 T.

Specific Absorbed Power

Some of the energy of RF radiation is absorbed by human tissue. *The specific absorbed power is the amount of RF energy absorbed per unit time per unit mass of tissue.* This is analogous to dose rate from ionizing radiations. The units are watts per kilogram (W/kg).

Specific Absorption Rate

This is the same as specific absorbed power.

Chapter 3
The Amount
of Radiation
Absorbed by the Conceptus

Ionizing Radiologic Modalities

It would be convenient if we could supply the reader with a table specifying the conceptus dose for all standard radiologic procedures. Unfortunately, this is not possible because dose to the conceptus of individual patients may vary by as much as a factor of 50 or more, depending on the radiographic equipment used, the size of the patient, and the methods used by the radiologist in performing the study. This is especially critical for studies involving the lower abdomen and pelvis.

On the other hand, it is not always necessary to know the exact dose delivered to the uterus of a patient in order to make prudent decisions regarding patient management. In these cases, it is necessary only to know that the dose did not exceed a certain level. In Table 3-1, we list some estimated upper-limit values of radiation that might be delivered to the uterus of a patient from various studies. These upper-limit values assume there is no direct exposure to the uterus from either radiography or fluoroscopy. The reader should be aware that the majority of studies will deliver significantly less quantities of radiation than the upper limits given in Table 3-1.

No dose value is given for lower abdominal radiographic and fluoroscopic studies since these doses are usually higher and can vary by considerable magnitudes. An upper-limit estimate would be of little use because the actual dose from such studies can be very small or very high. For example, a large patient might easily receive four to ten times more radiation than a thin patient. Fluoroscopy performed in an anteroposterior (AP) position as opposed to a posteroanterior (PA) position might result in a factor of 4 difference in conceptus dose. The amount of radiation required for the proper film darkening can vary by a factor of 10, depending on the type of equipment used. Because uterine dose depends on these parameters, it is not possible to provide the reader with a practical upper-limit estimate of dose received from these studies. For studies involving the lower abdomen, a more precise estimate of conceptus dose can be obtained from a radiological physicist. This is reviewed in Chapter 6.

Table 3-1. Upper-Limit Conceptus Dose from Selected X-Ray Examinations[a]

Examination	Dose
Routine head	< 50 mrad
Routine thoracic and neck	
Chest	< 50 mrad
Mammography	< 50 mrad
Cervical spine	< 50 mrad
Thoracic spine	< 100 mrad
Routine extremity	
Upper femur	(?)
Other (including shoulder and knee arthrography)	< 50 mrad
Routine pelvic	(?)
Angiography	
Cerebral	< 100 mrad
Cardiac catheterization	< 500 mrad
Aortography	< 100 mrad
Abdominal	(?)
Myleography	(?)
Gastrointestinal	(?)
Urologic	(?)
Computed tomography	
Head (single series of entire head at 1-cm slice intervals)	< 50 mrad
Chest (single series of entire chest at 1-cm slice intervals)	< 1 rad
Upper abdominal (20 1-cm consecutive slices more than 2.5 cm from uterus)	< 3 rad
Pelvic	(?)
Conventional tomography	
Head	< 100 mrad
Chest	< 500 mrad

[a]Assumes patient's pelvis is shielded or outside direct path of x-ray field. Doses can exceed these values if uterus is directly exposed or if x-ray field is not confined to anatomy of interest. A (?) means that an upper-limit estimate is not practical.

For radionuclide studies, the conceptus dose depends on the distribution of the radionuclide within the body of the patient. Table 3-5 provides estimates of the usual doses delivered from some radiopharmaceuticals. Many reasonable assumptions have been made in order to arrive at these estimates. Proper patient management requires that the uncertainties in dose evaluation be taken into account when quoting the values given in Table 3-5. These uncertainties are discussed later.

This chapter reviews radiographic and nuclear radiologic factors that influence conceptus dose. For diagnostic x rays, the imaging equipment is critical to evaluation of conceptus dose. The different types of equipment are reviewed along with other important factors such as variations in patient anatomy. In nuclear radiologic examinations, conceptus dose depends on the amount of radiopharmaceutical used and its distribution within the patient. In some situations, the type of equipment used in the study may influence the amount of radioactivity given, but this has only an indirect influence on patient dose and need not be reviewed here. Physiologic and metabolic factors do directly influence conceptus dose in nuclear radiologic studies, and these are reviewed.

Radiologists will be familiar with much of this material. Other physicians may find it useful because it reveals the complex nature of conceptus dose evaluation. Physicists commissioned with the task of dose evaluation will find that it reviews pitfalls and subtle aspects of the problem. Common assumptions, such as approximating the pregnant uterus to lie at central depth inside the pelvis, can result in significant miscalculations. The actual calculative procedures are described in Appendices A and B.

CONVENTIONAL RADIOGRAPHY

A conventional film-recorded radiographic examination is depicted in Figure 3-1. The highest radiation dose is delivered at the surface, where the x rays enter the patient. Some of the x rays are immediately absorbed by the tissue or are scattered away. In addition, there is backscattered radiation from tissues immediately beneath. Just below the surface, less radiation is available to interact in the tissues. By the time the x-ray beam reaches the uterus, the number of x rays is considerably reduced, and so the dose to the conceptus is much less than the surface dose. The amount of radiation energy absorbed by the conceptus depends on these factors: (1) the energy and number of x rays, (2) the depth of the conceptus, (3) patient positioning (*i.e.*, AP, PA, lateral, or oblique views), (4) the extent of the area exposed, (5) the proximity of the uterus to the anatomic area exposed, and (6) the number of films acquired. The importance of each of these factors and how each influences conceptus dose are discussed below.

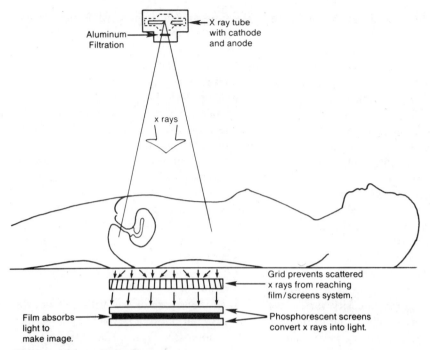

FIG. 3-1.   The standard radiograph.

The energy and number of x rays

Since the energies of x rays determine how easily they penetrate the patient, it is important to understand how various radiographic factors influence x-ray energy.

X rays are produced inside a glass vacuum tube (see Fig. 3-1), which houses a hot cathode and an anode. When high voltage is applied across the anode and cathode, electrons are stripped from the filament of the cathode and accelerated toward the anode. These electrons achieve high speeds and, upon collision with the anode, x rays with a wide range of energies are produced. The spectrum of x-ray energies is determined by the maximum, or peak, value and waveform of the kilovoltage as well as the materials between the anode and the patient.

The peak kilovoltage (kVp) across the x-ray tube generally varies from 60 kVp to 150 kVp for diagnostic x rays. (For some special applications, such as mammography, lower kVp techniques are used. Higher voltages are also occasionally employed for other examinations.)

Waveform refers to the time-dependent form in which the voltage is supplied to the x-ray tube. This may be a *single-phase* waveform or a *three-*

phase waveform. Single-phase is the type used in homes, while three-phase is commonly employed in industry. Each produces x rays with slightly different x-ray energy spectra.

The materials between the anode and the patient are the *filtration* and include intrinsic factors, such as the glass of the x-ray tube, and additional filter material, usually aluminum (see Fig. 3-1). The total filtration is normally specified as an aluminum equivalent, which is the amount of aluminum that, when placed in front of the x rays, would reduce their intensity to the same level as do the actual materials present. The equivalent quantity normally ranges from 0.5 mm to 4.5 mm of aluminum. Calculating conceptus dose at the wrong kVp, waveform, or filtration can result in inaccurate calculations.

The number of x rays incident on the patient is determined by kVp, waveform, and filtration as well as other important factors. These include the distance of the patient from the x-ray source, the sensitivity of the image-recording device (usually film), the patient's size, and the materials placed between the patient and the film, such as the table and grid (a device to help improve contrast on the radiograph).

X-ray intensity varies inversely with the square of the distance from the source. This is due to the fact that x rays fan out in an expanding sphere as they move away from their production point (see Figs. 1-1 and 3-1).

Various radiographic film systems require different amounts of radiation to produce a properly exposed film. The x rays themselves normally contribute to only a small fraction of the film blackening. The film is usually sandwiched between two "screens" made from a phosphorescent material that is activated by x rays (see Fig. 3-1). The light produced by the phosphor is proportional to the number of x rays striking it. Film is far more sensitive to light than to x rays. It is the light output from different areas of the phosphor screens that makes the major contribution to film blackening and creates the image. The light output of different phosphor screens per incident x ray varies considerably. The screen used depends on the image quality required for diagnosis. The conversion efficiency of photons to light can vary by a factor of 10 or more for commercially available screen–film combinations.

Thick patients attenuate substantially more x rays than thin patients do. The loss in x-ray penetration because of a thicker abdomen or pelvis must be compensated for by exposing the patient to more radiation. Thick patients may require up to 10 times more radiation than thin ones. Specific examples of patient size as an important consideration for dose calculations are given in Case Reports No. 2 and No. 3 of Chapter 11.

The table on which the patient lies absorbs some of the x rays. The material used in the manufacture of the tabletop can result in significant differences in dose. Conventional tabletops absorb 10% to 20% more x rays than carbon fiber tops absorb.

Grids are used to shield the film from scattered x rays that travel toward it (see Fig. 3-1). These scattered x rays expose the film, reduce the visibility of anatomic detail, and provide no diagnostic information. Only x rays that penetrate the patient without colliding with electrons will produce image detail. Because all grids prevent scattered x rays from reaching the film, there is a concomitant loss in film exposure, which must be compensated for by increasing radiation dose to the patient (usually by a factor of 2 to 8). Some grids are better at removing scatter radiation than others. Better grids yield better images at the cost of more dose to the patient.

Depth of the conceptus

Conceptus dose is dependent on conceptus depth, because tissues between the surface of the patient and the pregnant uterus attenuate the x-ray beam. The common assumption that the uterus lies half the AP distance inside the pelvis is not correct. Ragozzino and co-workers (1984) demonstrated in 16 randomly selected patients that the conceptus depth from the anterior surface in early pregnancy is about three tenths the AP thickness. Significant differences exist between the central and actual depth (Table 3-2). Furthermore, the uterus is not always in a forward position; it has a retroverted orientation in about 20% of all normal women (Parsons and Sommers, 1978).

The importance of this is illustrated by comparing results for conceptus dose from data of Gray and associates (1981) and Rosenstein (1976a, 1976b). Gray and associates measured uterine dose in a simulated human

Table 3-2. Conceptus Depth in Anteverted Uteri

Patient AP Thickness	Central Depth	Actual Conceptus Depth from Anterior Surface	Reference
19 cm[a]	9 cm[a]	6 cm[a]	Ragozzino and co-workers (1984)
26 cm	13 cm	6 cm	Wagner and co-workers (1983)
20 cm	10 cm	3.8 cm (bladder partially full) / 6.7 cm (bladder full)	Ragozzino and co-workers (1981)

[a]Average value of 16 early pregnancies

and assumed the uterus to be 12.0 cm from the anterior surface. Rosenstein calculated conceptus dose using a mathematical model assuming the depth to be 8.0 cm. For similar lower abdominal AP radiographic conditions, the uterine dose per entrance exposure in the two cases differed by about 200%. This disparity is explained in part by using the data of Harrison (1981), which show that the attenuation by 4 cm of tissue accounts for a factor of 2 difference in dose.

Conceptus depth is an especially significant factor when calculating conceptus dose from fluoroscopy. In conventional fluoroscopy, the beam enters the patient posteriorly (Fig. 3-2). If the uterus is anteverted, the conceptus will be exposed to less radiation than if it were at middistance. On the other hand, remote-control fluoroscopy delivers x rays anteriorly. In this case, dose to an anteverted uterus will be higher than the midline dose. The situation is reversed if the uterus is retroverted.

Two factors complicate the measurement of conceptus depth in early pregnancy: the distension of the bladder and the orientation of the patient (e.g., upright, supine, or prone). In one documented case, the depth of the gestational sac varied by 2.9 cm, depending on whether the bladder was partially filled or fully distended (see Table 3-2). The conceptus dose would differ by 40% in the two cases. This introduces an uncertainty into dose calculations that should be taken into consideration. Incorporating uncertainty of bladder distension into dose estimates is discussed in the section "Notes on Uncertainties" in Appendix A. An example of how conceptus depth can significantly influence conceptus dose is provided in Case Report No. 3 in Chapter 11.

Patient positioning

Conceptus dose depends significantly on whether the radiologic views acquired were AP, PA, lateral, or oblique. It is significant also to observe that in some cases, the conceptus may be somewhat shielded by anatomic parts (*e.g.*, maternal femur and pelvic wings in the lateral view).

Area exposed

The extent of the area exposed in the pelvis is a consideration because a large-area exposure produces a significant amount of scatter radiation from areas around the uterus. Some of this scatter reaches the conceptus. For small-area exposures, the percent of scatter radiation contributing to the total dose is reduced. An example of how significant field size can be in dose calculations is discussed in Appendix A, Example No. 2. Solution of this problem by Technique No. 2 yields a conceptus dose 40% too high because of too large a field size.

Proximity of the uterus to exposed areas

If the uterus is outside the area radiographed, the conceptus dose is limited to that delivered by scatter and leakage radiation. It drops off rapidly the farther the uterus is from the area radiographed (see Fig. A-10).

Number of films acquired

Finally, the total dose to a conceptus is the sum of doses for each film that was acquired. Repeating a single AP radiograph of the pelvis doubles the uterine dose.

FLUOROSCOPIC EXAMINATIONS

Dose to a conceptus from fluoroscopic examinations depends on several of the above factors, including energy of the x rays, the number of x-ray photons produced, the depth of the conceptus, patient positioning, area exposed, and the proximity of the uterus to the exposed areas. However, there are several additional factors peculiar to fluoroscopy (Fig. 3-2).

The geometry of conventional fluoroscopy is different from that of conventional radiography. The x-ray tube is beneath the table, and the image is displayed through an image intensifier placed above the patient. So-called *remote-control* fluoroscopy is done with x-ray tube above the patient and the image intensifier below the patient. Dose calculations for this device

FIG. 3-2. The fluoroscopic examination.

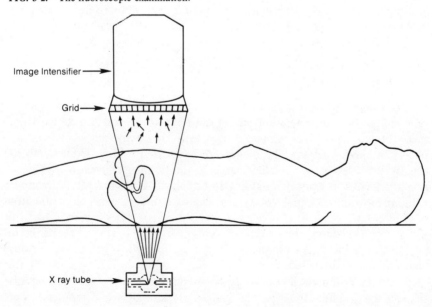

will be different from those for conventional fluoroscopy. The fluoroscopic x-ray rate is about 1% of the rate for radiographs, but the exposure to the patient lasts hundreds or thousands of times longer. The output rate and duration vary considerably from machine to machine and from examination to examination.

The x-ray output depends on the quality and design of the imaging system used to convert the x rays to a picture, usually displayed on a television screen. Some units have the option of varying (magnifying) the size of the image that appears on the screen. When the size of the image is magnified, the dose rate to the patient may increase by about a factor of 2 or more.

To estimate conceptus dose, these factors must be taken into account as well as others, including fluoroscopy kVp, whether or not a grid was used, and the duration of beam-on time. In addition, permanent images of the fluoroscopic examination are often acquired using radiographic spot-filming, 100-mm filming of the fluoroscopic image, and cine or video recordings. Contributions from these factors must be included to complete conceptus dose estimates.

Fluoroscopic examinations often involve the use of contrast agents, sometimes referred to as *dyes*. Anatomy that is coated by or filled with these materials is visually enhanced on the radiograph. Common contrast agents include air, barium sulfate, and iodinated organic materials. Air and barium sulfate are often used jointly to enhance the visibility of the gastro-intestinal tract. Organic iodinated compounds are administered orally, intravenously, or intra-arterially to enhance the vascular system, the urinary tract, and other areas. None of these agents emits radiation.

ANGIOGRAPHY

Conventional angiography employs fluoroscopic apparatus, but the geometric configuration and radiation output are often considerably different from those of standard fluoroscopic equipment. The x-ray output is usually pulsed in short bursts while images are recorded on film. The equipment usually provides more versatile maneuverability than conventional fluorographic devices, permitting anatomy to be looked at from several directions without moving the patient. A typical angiographic "C-arm" unit is shown in Figure 3-3.

DIGITAL SUBTRACTION ANGIOGRAPHY

Digital subtraction angiography uses apparatus similar to that in conventional angiography. However, the images are stored in a computer rather than on film. This permits the radiologist to enhance and manipulate the

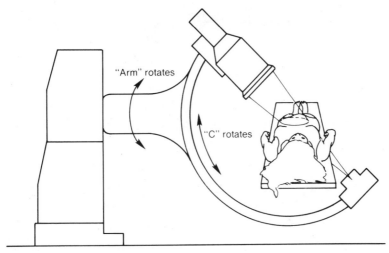

FIG. 3-3. A "C-arm" fluoroscopic unit.

data in order to extract information not available with conventional film. Since imaging regimens are different for computer-based studies versus film-based studies, doses to patients differ in the two cases. The actual dose depends on the regimen used.

CONVENTIONAL TOMOGRAPHY

Conventional tomography is a radiographic technique that employs a pivoting motion of the x-ray tube and screen–film system during the radiographic exposure (Fig. 3-4). This movement makes it possible to view anatomy at the level of the fulcrum, while blurring out anatomy above and below it. The geometry of such a device is different from that of conventional radiography because of this motion. If tomography of the abdomen is employed, doses to the patient can be significantly higher (up to a factor of 2 per film) than doses received for conventional abdominal films. Additionally, a large number of images exposing the same area are usually acquired. These factors must be taken into account when calculating dose to a conceptus. However, conventional tomography is usually used to study anatomy other than the pelvis. Therefore, most radiation received by a conceptus from such examinations would result from scatter and leakage radiation, not from primary radiation.

COMPUTED TOMOGRAPHY

Computed tomography (CT) uses entirely different configurations of x-ray tubes and detectors than does standard radiography, fluoroscopy, or con-

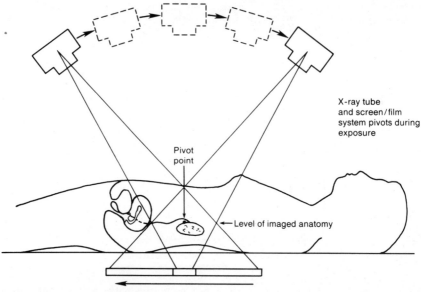

FIG. 3-4.   Conventional tomography.

ventional tomography. For this imaging system, an x-ray tube rotates around the patient, as shown in Figure 3-5. The transmission of the x-ray beam through the patient is recorded by detectors on the other side of the patient, and these data are stored in a computer. The x-ray beam has a very narrow fan shape covering only about a 1-cm width of the patient. Thus, for a single image, x rays are delivered from all sides of the patient, but only to a very narrow transaxial slice about 1-cm thick. Dose to the conceptus arising from examinations other than pelvic CT examinations will result from scatter and leakage radiation produced by this collimated beam. Typical doses to a conceptus from CT examinations distant from the uterus are very small. The actual dose depends on several factors, including the number of images that are acquired, the number of x rays used to create each image, the anatomic section scanned, and the type of machine used. Upper-limit estimates are provided in Table 3-1.

If the conceptus is in the direct path of the x-ray beam so that CT images of the uterus are obtained, then the conceptus dose from these CT scans is considerably greater than those from CT scans of other anatomic parts. Typically, because of overlying tissues, the dose to the middle of the patient is 70% ± 30% the surface dose. Since surface doses are on the order of 4 rad, the conceptus exposure from such a CT examination is between 1.6 rad and 4 rad. Caution is advised, since the precise dose depends on the machine and techniques used, the size of the patient, and so on.

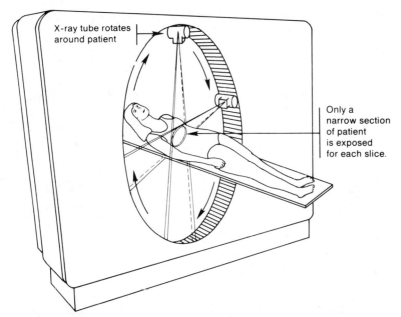

X-ray tube rotates
around patient

Only a
narrow section
of patient
is exposed
for each slice.

FIG. 3-5. Computed tomography.

One mistake often made is to assume incorrectly that doses from CT images are additive. For example, if the entrance dose from a single image (commonly called a slice) is 3 rad, it is incorrect to assume that the dose from 16 slices would be 48 rad. The total surface dose to the patient from such an examination might be from 3.6 rad to 5.4 rad. The reason for this is that the slices of the CT study lie side by side. Since each of these slices delivers approximately 3 rad to the surface of the patient, then, ideally, the total dose to the patient is only 3 rad to 16 different sections of her body. What has changed is the area exposed, which, instead of being 1-cm wide, is now 16-cm wide. Since the collimation of the x-ray beam is not perfect, there will be some radiation overlap from slice to consecutive slice. For this reason, the dose to the abdomen from a series of slices will be higher than that for a single slice, usually from 20% to 80% more.

CALCULATIONS OF ABSORBED X-RAY DOSE

Conceptus dose from routine extra-abdominal radiographic studies results only from scatter and leakage radiation. Under normal operating conditions, needed studies would not pose an unacceptable radiation risk. Table 3-3 reviews uterine doses from extra-abdominal radiography at a variety of diagnostic departments. These doses are less than the dose of about 50

Table 3-3.   Estimated Dose to Uterus from Extra-Abdominal Examinations[a]
(Fluoroscopic dose excluded)

Examination	Estimated Mean Dose (mrad/Examination)			Reported Range[e]
	BRH[b]	ICRP[c]	UNSCEAR[d]	
Dental		< 10	0.06	0.03 – 0.1
Head–cervical spine	< 0.5	< 10	< 10	< 0.5 – 3.0
Extremities	< 0.5	< 10	< 10	< 0.5 – 18.0
Shoulder	< 0.5	< 10		< 0.5 – 3.0
Thoracic spine	11	< 10		< 10 – 55
Chest (radiographic)	1		2	0.2 – 43
Chest (photofluorographic)	3	< 10	3	0.9 – 40
Mammography			< 10	
Femur (distal)		50	1	1 – 50

[a]NCRP (1977)
[b]BRH (1976)
[c]ICRP (1970)
[d]UNSCEAR (1972)
[e]Includes BRH (1976), ICRP (1970), UNSCEAR (1972), and Lindell and Dobson (1961)

mrem to 100 mrem received in 9 months from naturally occurring environmental radiation. Normally, it would be unnecessary to perform an in-depth conceptus dose evaluation for such studies because the dose is very small and would not be reason enough to alter patient management.

Abdominal examinations deliver considerably higher doses to the conceptus. A simple lookup table of nominal doses from such studies will not yield accurate dose evaluations and can render estimates that are grossly misleading. Table 3-4 lists uterine doses for abdominal radiography performed at a variety of diagnostic departments. Note that in the case of the intravenous pyelogram (IVP), the reported uterine dose varies from 70 mrad to 5500 mrad. (This dose does not include fluoroscopy.) The wide range dramatically demonstrates a need for careful evaluation in the management of pregnant patients.

Several techniques and plenty of data are available to assist in the calculation of conceptus dose once the information regarding the equipment used, the number of examinations conducted, the number of films made, and the techniques for both radiography and fluoroscopy used have been acquired (Ragozzino et al, 1981; Harrison, 1981; Säbel et al, 1980; Schulz and Gignac, 1976; Kelley and Trout, 1971). The technical and quantitative details of these methods are reviewed in Appendix A.

One technique often used to calculate conceptus dose is based on calculations using a mathematically modeled anatomic replica of the average female anatomy (Rosenstein, 1976a, 1976b). This technique is also reviewed

Table 3-4. **Estimated Dose to Uterus from Abdominal Examinations**[a]
(Fluoroscopic dose excluded)

Examination	Estimated Mean Dose (mrad/Examination)			
	BRH[b]	ICRP[c]	UNSCEAR[d]	Reported Range[e]
Upper GI series	171	150		5–1,230
Cholecystography Cholangiography	78	150	120	14–1,600
Lumbar spine	990	550	560	27–3,970
Lumbosacral spine			470	100–2,440
Pelvis	290	340	320	55–2,190
Hips and femur (proximal)	170	690	330	73–1,370
Urography, IV or	810	960	810	70–5,480
Retrograde pyleogram		1,100	715	120–5,480
Urethrocystography		2,060		275–4,110
Lower GI tract (barium enema)	1,240	1,100	1,200	28–12,600
Abdomen	300	690	290	25–1,920
Abdomen (obstetric)		1,370 (fetal)	410	150–2,200
Pelvimetry		5,480	850	220–5,480
Hysterosalpingography		1,650	1,740	270–9,180

[a]Adapted from NCRP (1977). All values are for radiography only (no fluoroscopy). Doses listed for lower abdominal studies are 37% higher than those in NCRP (1977). See NCRP (1977), p 9, footnote (a).
[b]BRH (1976)
[c]ICRP (1970)
[d]UNSCEAR (1972)
[e]Includes BRH (1976), ICRP (1970), UNSCEAR (1972), and Lindell and Dobson (1961)

in Appendix A. Such estimates are accurate only insofar as the patient undergoing the study is adequately described by the model. The author of this technique advises caution in the use of these tables for evaluation of individual doses in the introduction of his book entitled *Handbook of Selected Doses for Projections Common in Diagnostic Radiology.* Specifically he states that "assignment of organ doses to individual patients using the Handbook data is not recommended."

Methods to calculate dose when the conceptus is not in the direct path of the x-ray beam are also reviewed in Appendix A. Doses to the conceptus from scatter radiation resulting from examinations that do not include the uterus may be estimated using Figure A-10. Under normal operating conditions, if the dose to the conceptus is solely from leakage and scatter radiation, it would not, by itself, be of sufficient magnitude to warrant interruption of a pregnancy. It may, however, be of sufficient magnitude to consider postponing a study or performing only a limited examination on a patient known to be pregnant.

NUCLEAR RADIOLOGIC EXAMINATIONS

For these procedures, the radiation dose to the conceptus results from radionuclides introduced into the patient by injection or oral consumption. The dose is related entirely to the quantity, decay characteristics, and distribution dynamics of radiopharmaceuticals introduced. Because the imaging equipment is not the source of the radiation, it is not necessary to have an understanding of imaging techniques or radiation detection instrumentation as was necessary for x-ray imaging.

The dose to the developing child from radioisotopes introduced into the mother can be separated into doses from radionuclides in (1) maternal organs, (2) the placenta, and (3) the embryo/fetus.

Conceptus dose from radionuclides in maternal organs or in the placenta arise only from gamma and x-radiations that penetrate the distance from the organ to the developing child. There will be no beta (electron or positron) radiation dose from tissues external to the unborn child because this radiation is not penetrating (*i. e.*, it travels less than 1 mm in tissue). It does not traverse the tissues separating the source organ from the developing child.

Radionuclides that cross the placenta and enter into the organs of the embryo or fetus can give rise to significantly higher doses. In this setting, substantial doses can be delivered by isotopes emitting nonpenetrating radiations, since the embryonic or fetal organs will absorb all their energy.

The factors to consider in evaluating conceptus and embryonic or fetal doses include: (1) the amount of radioactivity administered; (2) the concentrations of the radioactivity in the various organs of the body; (3) the proximity of each of these organs to the conceptus; (4) the particular types of radiation the radionuclide emits; (5) the amount of radiopharmaceutical that crosses the placenta and enters into the embryo or fetus; (6) the conception age; (7) the length of time the radionuclides spend in each of the organs of the body, which, in turn, depends on the physical half-life of the radionuclide and the ability of the organ to eliminate the radiopharmaceutical.

Amount of radioactivity administered

The radiation dose to a developing child from a radionuclide procedure is directly proportional to the amount of radioactivity injected into the patient. The amount of radioactivity used in a study depends on the radiopharmaceutical, the type of study, and the age and size of the patient in the case of adolescents. Records of the amount of radioactivity administered should be available from the department performing the examination.

Concentrations of radioactivity in organs

Conceptus dose from radioactivity in an organ depends on how much radioactivity is in the organ. The concentration of radionuclides in tissues is governed by several factors, including the type of radiopharmaceutical used and the functional status of the organs.

Proximity of organs to the developing child

The dose from radioactivity concentrated in maternal organs is much less for distant organs than for organs close to the uterus. This is because the radiation spreads out, becoming less intense with increased distance from its source, and because the developing child is better shielded from the radioactivity with increased amounts of tissue separating the source organ from the uterus.

Type of radiation

As previously discussed in Chapter 1, the radiation dose received by a conceptus depends on the types of radiations released by the radionuclide. For concentrations in maternal organs and the placenta, the most important radiations contributing to the dose to the unborn child are gamma and x-ray photons. The energies of these photons determine how easily they penetrate the tissues separating the source organ from the conceptus. For radionuclides concentrating within the developing child, all types of radiations, including gamma rays, x rays, beta particles, and atomic electrons, must be considered in dose calculations.

Placental transfer of radiation

Limited data are available on the placental transfer of radiopharmaceuticals to the developing conceptus. It is known that with the use of some radiopharmaceuticals, specifically free iodine and iron 59, relative concentrations in the organs of the developing conceptus can be greater than those in the mother (see Chap. 1).

Conception age

The conception age is important in evaluating dose for two reasons. First, the relative position of the conceptus with respect to various organs will change as the conceptus grows. Second, conceptus maturity will govern the concentration of some radiopharmaceuticals within its own organs. For example, free iodine concentrates in the thyroid gland of the conceptus in amounts dependent on its developmental age (Dyer and Brill, 1969).

Length of time the radionuclide remains in the patient

The amount of time that the radiopharmaceutical remains in the patient depends on two factors. The first is the physical half-life of the radionuclide that is used to label the pharmaceutical. The second is the elimination of the radiopharmaceutical from each organ of the patient and her conceptus (the biologic half-life). This latter aspect depends on many factors. The function of the organ is one. For example, when analyzing kidney function with DTPA labeled with ^{99m}Tc, a healthy kidney will eliminate the DTPA in a relatively short time and transfer the activity to the urinary bladder. If there is a blockage in the urinary tract or altered renal function, the activity can be retained in the kidney. Dose to the conceptus in the two circumstances would be different. Additionally, the patient can govern the amount of time the radioactivity remains in her by the frequency with which she voids the radioactive urine. The patient should be advised to drink plenty of fluids and to void frequently for several days, commensurate with the type of radiopharmaceutical used. In this way, if she is pregnant, radioactivity is removed from her body as quickly as possible through the urinary tract, and the radiation dose to the conceptus from the nearby radioactivity within the bladder is reduced.

CALCULATIONS OF ABSORBED DOSE FROM RADIONUCLIDES

Conceptus dose calculations from radionuclide studies are only approximations. This results from the considerable uncertainties about the uptake of the radiopharmaceutical by individual maternal organs, the metabolism of the pharmaceutical by the patient, the proximity of these organs to the conceptus, and the placental uptake and transfer of the radionuclide. Available data are usually restricted to the average-size adult patient whose metabolism is modeled to represent the nonpregnant human (Snyder et al, 1978; Berman, 1977; Wooten, 1983).

For radionuclides excreted through the bladder, assumptions are made as to how much radioactivity is present as a function of time. This depends on the efficiency of the urinary tract and frequency of urination. Since the bladder is in contact with the uterus, these variations greatly complicate the dose to the conceptus from penetrating x and gamma radiations.

Most published dose calculations either do not account for conceptus uptake, or they assume the uptake to be the same as the general distribution of the radionuclide in the body of the mother (Hŭsák and Wiedermann, 1980; Smith and Warner, 1976). Wegst and associates (1984), Hahn and associates (1977, 1978), Mahon and associates (1973), Lathrop and associates (1976), and Dyer and Brill (1969) have studied placental uptake and transfer of radioactivity from some pharmaceuticals in rats, rabbits, mice, and humans. Extrapolation of findings in animals to application for humans is burdened with considerable uncertainty.

Table 3-5 lists the estimated dose to a conceptus per millicurie activity administered to the mother, based on an "average" patient. Assumptions regarding placental uptake of the pharmaceutical are noted. For pharmaceuticals known to cross the placenta (*i.e.,* ^{99m}Tc pertechnetate, free iodine, and ^{59}Fe) several authors have estimated the conceptus dose on the basis of data derived from animal or human investigations. For ^{99m}Tc pertechnetate,

Table 3-5. Conceptus Dose Estimates from Radiopharmaceuticals

Radiopharmaceutical	Conception Age (weeks)	Conceptus Organ	Dose Per Unit of Maternally Administered Activity (rad/mCi)	Footnotes
^{99m}Tc DTPA	1.5–6	Whole body	0.035	a
^{113m}In DTPA	1.5–6	Whole body	0.035	a
^{99m}Tc gluconate	1.5–6	Whole body	0.034	a
^{99m}Tc sodium pertechnetate	1.5–6	Whole body	0.027	a
^{99m}Tc sodium pertechnetate	1.5–6	Whole body	0.037	b,c
^{99m}Tc sodium pertechnetate	1.5–6	Whole body	0.039	b,d
^{99m}Tc sodium pertechnetate	<8	Whole body	0.048–0.32	e
^{99m}Tc polyphosphate	1.5–6	Whole body	0.025	a
^{99m}Tc sulfur colloid	1.5–6	Whole body	0.007	a,b
^{123}I sodium iodide	1.5–6	Whole body	0.032	b,f
^{131}I sodium iodide	1.5–6	Whole body	0.10	b,f
^{131}I sodium iodide	1.5–6	Whole body	0.15	a
^{131}I sodium iodide	7–9	Whole body	0.88	g,h
^{131}I sodium iodide	11	Whole body	1.15	g,i
^{131}I sodium iodide	12–13	Whole body	1.58	g,j
^{131}I sodium iodide	20	Whole body	3.00	g,i
^{131}I sodium iodide	11	Thyroid	715	g,i
^{131}I sodium iodide	12–13	Thyroid	1338	g,k
^{131}I sodium iodide	20	Thyroid	5900	g,f
^{123}I sodium rose bengal	1.5–6	Whole body	0.13	b
^{131}I sodium rose bengal	1.5–6	Whole body	0.68	b
^{67}Ga citrate	1.5–6	Whole body	0.25	a,l
^{75}Se methionine	1.5–6	Whole body	3.8	a
^{59}Fe citrate	7–20	Whole body	38	g,m
^{59}Fe citrate	7–13	Liver	410	g,n
^{59}Fe citrate	20	Liver	330	g,i
^{59}Fe citrate	11	Spleen	61.2	g,i
^{59}Fe citrate	12–13	Spleen	140	g,j
^{59}Fe citrate	20	Spleen	186	g,i

[a]Hüsák and Wiedermann (1980), assumes no uptake of activity in embryo
[b]Smith and Warner (1976), assumes activity distribution in embryo same as whole-body distribution in parent
[c]Resting population
[d]Nonresting population
[e]Wegst and co-workers (1984), accounts for placental uptake and transfer of radiopharmaceutical to embryo/fetus based on 15-day gestation rats
[f]Assumes 15% uptake in maternal thyroid
[g]Dyer and Brill (1969), dose estimates from human aborti
[h]Average value of 2 cases
[i]Value of 1 case
[j]Average value of 5 cases
[k]Average value of 4 cases
[l]Wegst and co-workers (1975) suggest that fetal self-irradiation from gallium 67 is not significant compared to fetal dose from concentration in maternal organs and placenta
[m]Average value of 9 cases
[n]Average value of 8 cases

whole-body conceptus dose estimates range from 0.023 rad per millicurie administered to 0.32 rad per millicurie. This latter estimate is based on an extrapolation of 15-day-old rat conceptuses, and the accuracy of such extrapolations is questionable. For free iodine, human data indicate the dose increases considerably as gestation progresses. Note that doses to individual organs of the conceptus are considerably higher than the whole-body conceptus dose for ^{131}I and [59]Fe.

In Appendix B, calculations required to estimate conceptus dose in general circumstances are reviewed.

Nonionizing Modalities

ULTRASOUND

An accurate evaluation regarding the amount of energy transferred to a conceptus from ultrasound examination is impossible. It is unnecessary in view of the lack of definitive evidence that there is any harm to a conceptus from such studies. This should not lead to a false sense of security regarding the safety of this technique. Ultrasound is a medical procedure from which the patient potentially derives a health benefit. Diagnostic ultrasound has been shown to induce biologic effects *in vitro* (see Chap. 1), but the significance of such observations is not known. We recommend that it not be used for other than medically indicated purposes. Studies on pregnant women should be limited to the amount of time required to obtain satisfactory information. Thus, any potential risks can be minimized.

MAGNETIC RESONANCE

The important quantities for assessing possible biologic risks from magnetic resonance (MR) are (1) magnetic-field strength, (2) time dependence and magnitude of the changing magnetic-field gradients, and (3) the specific absorbed power from the radiofrequency radiation. The magnetic-field strength is a well-known quantity for each MR imager. The time dependence and magnitude of the changing magnetic-field gradients depend on the pulse sequence used in imaging. The specific absorbed power depends on the pulse sequence and the size of the patient. Some estimates of this quantity have been made (see Budinger, 1981; or Mansfield and Morris, 1982). Since at this time there is very little information regarding potential biologic effects on conceptuses from MR, this information is of little value in patient management.

The foregoing remarks do not mean that MR imaging of pregnant women should not be approached cautiously. As of this writing, we are aware of only limited published results examining the biologic effects of

MR on pregnant animals. Since MR is in a rapid state of development, we anticipate that more data will appear in the near future. At this time, we caution against its use in pregnant women until its efficacy and safety are established by animal studies.

References

Berman M: Kinetic Models for Absorbed Dose Calculations, MIRD pamphlet No. 12. New York, Society of Nuclear Medicine, 1977

Budinger TF: Nuclear magnetic resonance (NMR) *in vivo* studies: Known thresholds for health effects. J Comput Assist Tomogr 5:800, 1981

BRH (Bureau of Radiological Health): Gonad Doses and Genetically Significant Dose from Diagnostic Radiology, US 1964 and 1970, DHEW publication (FDA) 76-8034. Rockville, MD, US Department of Health, Education, and Welfare, 1976

Dyer NC, Brill AB: Fetal radiation dose from maternally administered ^{59}Fe and [131]I. In Sikov MR, Mahlum DD (eds): Radiation Biology of the Fetal and Juvenile Mammal, pp 73–88. Oak Ridge, Tennessee, USAEC Division of Technical Information, 1969

Gray JE, Ragozzino MW, Van Lysel MS et al: Normalized organ doses for various diagnostic radiologic procedures. Am J Roent 137:463, 1981

Hahn K, Brod KH, Wolf R et al: Untersuchungen zur strahlenbelastung des feten bei nuklearmedizinischen untersuchungen von graviden. In Nuklearmedizin. Qualitatskriterien in der Nuklearmedizin. Stuttgart, New York, FK Schattauer, 1977

Hahn K, Wolf R, Eissner D: Die Strahlenbelastung des Foeten bei nuklearmedizinischen untersuchungen von graviden. Vortrag beim Inter. Rontgenkongress. Rio de Janeiro, 1978

Harrison RM: Central-axis depth-dose data for diagnostic radiology. Phys Med Biol 26:657, 1981

Hüsák V, Wiedermann M: Radiation absorbed dose estimates to the embryo from some nuclear medicine procedures. Eur J Nucl Med 5:205, 1980

ICRP (International Commission on Radiological Protection): Protection of the Patient in X-Ray Diagnosis, publication 16. Oxford, Pergamon Press, 1970

Kelley JP, Trout ED: Physical characteristics of the radiation from 2-pulse, 12-pulse, and 1000-pulse x-ray equipment. Radiology 100:653, 1971

Lathrop KA, Gloria IV, Harper PV: Response of mouse fetus to radiation from Na-99m-TcO$_4$. Biological and Environmental Effects of Low-Level Radiation, Proc Symp Chicago, Vol II, p 211. Vienna, IAEA, 1976

Lindell B, Dobson RL: Ionizing Radiation and Health, Public Health Papers, No. 6. Geneva, World Health Organization, 1961

Mahon DF, Subramanian G, McAfee JG: Experimental comparison of radioactive agents for studies of the placenta. J Nucl Med 14:651, 1973

Mansfield P, Morris PG: NMR Imaging in Biomedicine, pp 297–332. New York, Academic Press, 1982

NCRP (National Council on Radiation Protection and Measurements): Medical Radiation Exposure of Pregnant and Potentially Pregnant Women, report No. 54. Washington, DC, National Council on Radiation Protection and Measurements, 1977

Parsons CL, Sommers SC: Gynecology, 2nd ed, p 1437, Philadelphia, WB Saunders, 1978

Ragozzino MW, Breckle R, Hill LM et al: Average fetal depth *in utero*: Data for estimation of fetal absorbed dose from radiographic examinations, 1984. (in press)

Ragozzino MW, Gray JE, Burke TM et al: Estimation and minimization of fetal absorbed dose: Data from common radiographic examinations. Am J Roent 137:667, 1981

Rosenstein M: Organ Doses in Diagnostic Radiology, HEW publication (FDA) 76-8030. Rockville, Maryland, Bureau of Radiological Health, 1976a

Rosenstein M: Handbook of Selected Organ Doses for Projections Common in Diagnostic Radiology, HEW publication (FDA) 76-8031. Rockville, Maryland, Bureau of Radiological Health, 1976b

Säbel M, Bednar W, Weishaar J: Investigation of the exposure to radiation of the embryo/fetus in the course of radiographic examinations during pregnancy. 1st communication: Tissue–air ratios for X-rays with tube voltages between 60 kV and 120 kV. Strahlentherapie 156:502, 1980

Schulz RJ, Gignac C: Application of tissue–air ratios for patient dosage in diagnostic radiology. Radiology 120:687, 1976

Smith EM, Warner GG: Estimates of radiation dose to the embryo from nuclear medicine procedures. J Nucl Med 17:836, 1976

Snyder WS, Ford MR, Warner GG: Estimates of Specific Absorbed Fractions for Photon Sources Uniformly Distributed in Various Organs of a Heterogeneous Phantom, MIRD pamphlet No. 5 (revised). New York, Society of Nuclear Medicine, 1978

UNSCEAR (United Nations Scientific Committee on the Effects of Atomic Radiation): Ionizing Radiation, Levels and Effects, Vol. 1. New York, United Nations, 1972

Wagner LK, Lester RG, Schull WJ: Diagnostic radiation and the pregnant patient. Radiology 149(P):275, 1983

Wegst AV, Goin JE, Robinson RG: Cumulated activities determined from biodistribution data in pregnant rats ranging from 13 to 21 days. I. Tc-99m pertechnetate. Med Phys 10:841, 1984

Wegst AV, Robinson RG, Riley RC: Transplacental transfer of Ga-67. J Nucl Med 16:581, 1975

Wooten WW: Radionuclide kinetics in MIRD dose calculations. J Nucl Med 24:621, 1983

Chapter 4
Prenatal Risks from Ionizing Radiations, Ultrasound, Magnetic Fields, and Radiofrequency Waves

Ionizing Radiations

SOURCES OF DATA ON BIOEFFECTS

Reasonably suspected risks include resorption of the conceptus, nonrecoverable growth retardation, small head size, malformation, mental retardation, and childhood cancer. Information regarding the effects of radiation on conceptuses is derived from animal studies, human exposures to diagnostic radiation, human exposures to therapeutic radiation, and human exposures to atomic bomb radiation at Hiroshima and Nagasaki. Many reviews are available (BEIR, 1980; Brent and Gorson, 1972a; Brent, 1972b, 1977, 1980, 1983; Hoffman, 1981; Rugh, 1958; Sternberg, 1973; Tabuchi, 1964; Nokkentved, 1968; UNSCEAR, 1984; Villumsen, 1970; Yamazaki, 1966).

Animal data are used to study radiation effects under controlled conditions. Care must be exercised when extrapolating from animal data to possible consequences for humans.

Human exposures to diagnostic x rays have been associated with isolated cases of malformation, but causality is highly speculative. Epidemiologic studies have correlated diagnostic x rays with small increases in the incidence of childhood cancer. Although more compelling than the malformation data, this effect is also controversial because of difficulties in proving the radiation was a causal agent.

Therapeutic exposures to radiation have definitely caused malformations. However, direct extrapolation of effects observed at therapeutic levels to effects at diagnostic levels has dubious value.

Much of our information regarding malformation is derived from the exposure of the large populations at Hiroshima and Nagasaki. Over 2800 pregnant women were exposed at the 2 sites. Over 500 conceptuses received more than 1 rad of radiation. The children of these women have been studied in relation to the amount of radiation they received and their conception age when exposed. The reported dose levels are controversial, and it is not certain whether neutron radiation at Hiroshima was significant (Kerr et al, 1983). These factors and the environmental conditions following these tragedies introduce uncertainty into the dose–effect relationship and whether or not the observed effects were caused solely by the radiation.

DOSE DEPENDENCE

Diagnostic levels of radiations may or may not cause perceptible deleterious effects on unborn children. If such effects occur, they are sporadic and infrequent events. It is not possible to predict whether an exposed conceptus will suffer a radiation-induced anomaly. The best we can do is draw on past experience and state, based on our best estimations, the likelihood that an abnormality might occur.

The probability of causing deleterious effects depends on the amount of radiation delivered. The manner in which the risk increases with increased dose is not always known. In Figures 4-1, 4-2, and 4-3, three possibilities are shown. The linear-no-threshold theory (see Fig. 4-1) holds that increased risk is zero only at zero dose, and it increases linearly as dose increases. In this model, it is assumed that any amount of radiation, no matter how small, proportionately increases the likelihood that the child will be affected. In the linear-threshold model (see Fig. 4-2), it is postulated there is a dose below which no effect occurs and above which the risk of in-

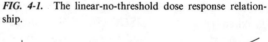

FIG. 4-1. The linear-no-threshold dose response relationship.

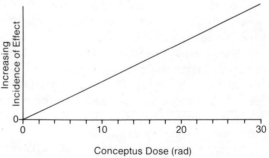

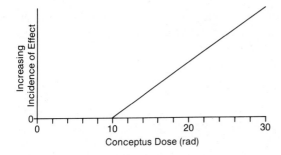

FIG. 4-2. The linear-threshold dose response relationship.

ducing the deleterious effect increases linearly. The linear-quadratic model (see Fig. 4-3) assumes a relationship that falls between the previous two. The elevated incidence increases slightly at very low doses, rising more steeply with larger ones. Data on human conceptus exposures indicate that, for some effects, the linear-no-threshold model applies, while for other effects, the other models apply. (Some readers may be familiar with a dose-response curve that turns over at high doses, showing a decreasing incidence of an effect with increasing dose from cell killing. This effect is not relevant to diagnostic levels of radiation.)

DOSE RATE DEPENDENCE

Radiation-induced effects depend not only on the dose, but also on the rate at which the dose is delivered. In circumstances where the dose is delivered at low rates over long periods of time, repair mechanisms can compensate for the damage produced by the radiation. However, if the damage occurs too rapidly, the repair mechanisms are not capable of keeping up with the damage, and a deleterious effect is more likely to result, even though the cumulative dose in the two circumstances may have been identical. This is

FIG. 4-3. The linear-quadratic dose response relationship.

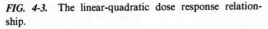
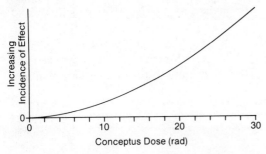

relevant when considering the effects that may result from multiple diagnostic studies extended over a period of time or from radionuclide studies where the dose is distributed over many days.

MALFORMATION AND PRENATAL DEATH

Prenatal Death

Recent studies have estimated that between 35% and 62% of all human pregnancies do not reach viability. Of these, the vast majority abort without interruption of the regular menstrual cycle (Edmonds et al, 1982; Miller et al, 1980). From animal data, Brent and Gorson (1972a) have shown that radiation-induced prenatal death (resorption) might occur at doses as low as 10 rad if delivered prior to implantation. These data suggest that radiation-induced resorption at doses lower than this is highly unlikely. Because of the lack of human data, no detailed dose-response relationship is available. The risk to the mother in this case is generally small, since an abortion of this nature goes undetected and may manifest itself only as a missed menstrual period.

After implantation, radiation-induced prenatal death occurs at other stages of gestation only at much higher dose levels (25 rad), that is, beyond the usual diagnostic realm.

Growth impairment

Wood and associates (1967) demonstrated that *in utero* doses to Japanese A-bomb victims resulted in impaired growth for children followed through age 17. Subjects within 1500 meters of the blast were, on the average, 2 cm to 3 cm shorter, about 3 kg lighter, and had 1 cm smaller head circumference than normal. No correlation with gestation age was evident. The conceptus dose for the group of subjects within 1500 meters from the center of the blast was greater than 25 rad (Kerr et al, 1983). However, the height, weight, and head size were generally normal for those exposed beyond 1500 meters. These latter subjects were exposed to radiation levels less than 25 rad. Although these negative results at less than 25 rad are encouraging, they do not prove that all effects are negative. Refined studies (see below) and improved dose information might alter these conclusions.

Small head size

Miller and Blot (1972) and Miller and Mulvihill (1976) examined the correlation of small head size (SHS)* with dose to the mother and gestation

---

*Head circumference was said to be small if in one or more examinations from 10 to 19 years it was at least two standard deviations below the average for the age or sex of the patient in each city, and was on all previous and subsequent examinations at least one standard deviation below the average.

age. Small head size is often referred to as *microcephaly*. The literature in this case is somewhat misleading in that microcephaly often carries an implication of mental retardation. This is not the case for SHS in these studies. Only about 20% of the subjects with SHS were classified as mentally retarded. At Hiroshima, SHS was most prevalent if exposure occurred between 2 and 15 weeks postconception. The increased incidence of SHS during this period was about 1% per rad delivered to the conceptus for doses comparable to diagnostic levels (< 10 rad). However, whether or not radiation was the sole cause of this effect is uncertain. Miller and Mulvihill state, "In Nagasaki no effect was demonstrable under 150 rad (mother's dose, approximately 75-rad conceptus dose). The number of intrauterine exposures there, though substantially fewer than Hiroshima, was ample to show an effect comparable to that in Hiroshima, had there been one." Other compounding factors (*e.g.*, nutritional) might have been involved at Hiroshima.*

Severe mental retardation

As pointed out previously, rapid neuron development of the cerebral hemispheres occurs during the 8th through 16th weeks postconception (Dobbing and Sands, 1973). Mole (1982) reported that the incidence of radiation-induced severe mental retardation (SMR)[†] in the *in utero* Japanese A-bomb survivors was greatest during this period. Otake and Schull (1984) combined the data from Nagasaki and Hiroshima to show that the incidence of SMR for exposures during the 8th through 15th weeks postconception was about 0.4% per rad delivered to the fetus.[‡] The data are consistent with the linear-no-threshold model for risk assessment. However, there was no increased incidence of SMR at doses less than 1 rad. The incidence associated with *in utero* exposures occurring between the 16th and 25th weeks postconception was about 0.2% per rad but was evident only at doses greater than 50 rad. For this gestation time, the linear-threshold model may be applicable, with the threshold at approximately 50 rad.

Again, it is questionable whether or not radiation was a cause or the sole cause of this effect. Evidence that it may not have been includes nonradiation-related health problems that might account for some SMR cases, and the fact that there was no increase in SMR for the 23 subjects exposed

---

*Prior to 1980, it had been thought that the neutron dose at Hiroshima was responsible for this disparity in effect at the two cities. It is now thought that the neutron dose at Hiroshima was too small to account for it (Kerr et al, 1983).

[†]Children were classified as severely mentally retarded if they were "unable to perform simple calculations, to make simple conversation, to care for oneself, or if he or she was completely unmanageable or had to be institutionalized." (Otake and Schull, 1984)

[‡]The most recent (prior to February 1984) data on dose estimates would not significantly alter the conclusions made here.

to conceptus doses up to 100 rad at Nagasaki during the 8th through 15th weeks postconception.

There was no elevation in SMR for subjects exposed up to 100 rad during any other time of gestation at either Hiroshima or Nagasaki.

Other forms of malformations

There is a conspicuous paucity of information citing externally administered ionizing radiation as a causal agent for other types of malformation in humans. Brent (1980) has pointed out that "no . . . bonafide radiation-induced morphological malformation has been reported in a human that has not exhibited growth retardation or central nervous system abnormality." Mole (1982) further noted that "there is nothing positive in support of the belief that early stages of human development are sensitive to induction of malformations by relatively large radiation doses, let alone to the much smaller doses characteristic of . . . radiologic examinations in medicine."

The previous paragraph applies to externally administered radiation. For internally administered radiation, the metabolism of the radiopharmaceutical may cause high concentrations of the radionuclide in organs of a conceptus if the material crosses the placenta. This may result in dysfunctioning fetal organs. The classic example of this effect involves the use of ^{131}I after the eighth week postconception (Stoffer and Hamburger, 1976). Iodine concentrates in the fetal thyroid in amounts considerably greater than those in the maternal thyroid (see Table 3-5). Hypothyroidism results from large doses of ^{131}I to the fetal thyroid.

Congenital malformation from diagnostic x rays

If a child is born with a birth defect, and the mother had received a diagnostic radiologic study while pregnant, speculation about cause and effect frequently ensues. Such speculation can only raise questions or suspicions, but it would be imprudent and rash to hasten to conclusions. These anecdotal observations cannot always take into account certain events that could explain the incident. For example, the mother may have been taking teratogenic drugs or may have had a viral infection or another problem that could account for the defect. There may be a genetic reason for the problem, or the x-ray study may have been requested because of complications that led to the defect. The relationship between the x rays and the defects may merely be a coincidence, not one of cause and effect. There are a few reports that correlate birth defects with radiation (Heinonen et al, 1977; Jacobsen and Mellemgaard, 1968; Hammer-Jacobsen, 1959). Although these reports cautiously raise questions of possible teratogenic effects of x rays, they are inconclusive. Several retrospective and prospective studies have attempted to investigate rigorously the correlation of diagnostic x rays with birth defects. These are summarized in the following paragraphs.

In a retrospective study, Tabuchi (1964) found a 1.4% incidence of deformities in 2220 children exposed to low doses of radiation (less than 1 rad in 83% of the cases and greater than 5 rad in 0.5% of the cases). This was slightly higher than the 0.7% incidence of deformities in the nonexposed group. The greatest frequency of deformity occurred in 117 children exposed prior to the third month of gestation (4 of 117, or 3.4%). However, the pregnancies involving deformed children were also complicated by other factors that had been associated with birth defects more often than were the pregnancies involving normal children. These factors included genital bleeding, medications, and a previous history of birth defects. They could account for some of the incidence in the exposed group. The radiation was therefore not suspected as a cause of the increase.

Villumsen (1970) prospectively studied 3157 pregnancies involving women exposed to diagnostic x-ray examination. Unfortunately, no dosimetry is available. Forty-four women were exposed to abdominal radiography in the first trimester. There was no indication of an increased incidence of small head size. One child was malformed. The birth defect, congenital heart disease, was not thought to be linked with the exposure because it occurred at a stage in pregnancy later than is necessary to cause the defect. Seven hundred eighty-five of the exposed women had abdominal studies in the second and third trimesters. There was no significant increase in malformation in these cases. There was also no increase among the children of the remaining women, who received only extra-abdominal studies.

One hundred fifty-two children of mothers exposed to abdominal examinations during the first four months of pregnancy were studied by Nokkentved (1968). No dosimetry was performed, but the doses were probably less than 5 rad and perhaps on the order of hundreds of millirads. There was no evidence of teratogenic effects. There was a small increase in the incidence of growth retardation when exposure occurred during the second month of gestation, but this incidence was not statistically conclusive.

In a study involving 1199 subjects, Kinlen and Acheson (1968) retrospectively found no correlation between congenital malformation and prenatal exposure to diagnostic radiation during the first trimester. However, only two of the subjects received abdominal radiography. Because of the low doses received from chest, head, and extremity radiography, no radiation-induced effect would be anticipated, and thus the results are not surprising.

A matched-pair study investigating central nervous system (CNS) defects in Finland was undertaken by Granroth (1979) to determine if there could be a link with diagnostic x-ray examinations. This study included 710 children with CNS defects and 710 without such defects. No dosimetry is available. Only 9 mothers in the study received abdominal radiography in the first trimester, whereas 282 had abdominal studies during the second and third trimesters. The remainder received chest x rays or pelvic x rays prior to pregnancy. There were a few associations between congenital defects of the CNS and diagnostic x-ray examinations, but the associations were either statistically insignificant, or the defects themselves may have been the reasons the diagnostic x-ray studies were requested.

A retrospective matched-pair study investigating the correlation between diagnostic x rays and neural tube defects was reported by Choi and Klaponski (1970). No dosimetry is reported, and there is no description of the types of studies performed. No correlation between x rays and neural tube defects was found.

These investigations indicate that, if there is a risk for malformation from diagnostic x-ray studies, it is small. However, it would be rash to conclude that there are no risks. The actual number of abdominal exposures resulting in modest conceptus doses (more than 1 rad) of diagnostic radiation during critical periods of pregnancy are too few in number. This renders any conclusions inapplicable for women receiving higher conceptus doses at times when the conceptus is sensitive to radiation induced defects. We can conclude, however, that any increased incidence of malformation from very low doses (less than 1 rad) of diagnostic radiation during pregnancy is so small as to go undetected by these studies.

MALIGNANCIES

Stewart and Kneale (1970) and Kneale and Stewart (1976a, 1976b) demonstrated a correlation between an increased incidence of childhood cancer and *in utero* doses of about 2 rad. Several other studies have corroborated this association of prenatal exposure to x rays and increased likelihood of childhood cancers (MacMahon, 1962; Diamond et al, 1973; Graham et al, 1966; Monson and MacMahon, 1984). Other data suggest that radiation has a dubious causal relationship with cancer (Court-Brown et al, 1960; Jablon and Kato, 1970). The carcinogenicity of *in utero* diagnostic radiation continues to be a matter for debate. We conservatively assume that the risk established by Stewart and Kneale represents an upper-limit estimate of the true risk.

They specified that under normal circumstances 99.93% of the children in Great Britain did not develop cancer. If exposed during the first trimester, the relative increase in cancer per rad is 250% (BEIR, 1980). If exposed during the second or third trimester, the relative increase per rad is 64% (BEIR, 1980). These percent increases often contribute to misconceptions about the absolute risk as discussed in this text's Introduction. A different and more meaningful perspective is provided in Table 4-1, where, based on the above risks, we list the likelihood the child will not contract the disease.

Table 4-1. *Percent of Likelihood of Not Developing Childhood Cancer After Prenatal Diagnostic Irradiation*

Gestation Age	Conceptus Dose			
	0 rad	1 rad	5 rad	10 rad
1st Trimester	99.93%	99.75%	99.12%	98.25%
2nd or 3rd Trimester	99.93%	99.88%	99.70%	99.48%

GENETIC MUTATIONS AND STERILITY

Little is known about radiation-induced genetic defects that might be transferred to the progeny of children exposed *in utero.* The BEIR Committee (1980) report suggests that the mutational sensitivity of early male germline cells is not very different from that of spermatogonia. The early germline cells in the fetal oogonia are perhaps 1.6 times more radiosensitive than mature oocytes after birth. This makes them about as sensitive as spermatogonia. Therefore, the female fetal gonads are perhaps slightly more sensitive than adult gonads. To try to gain some perspective on the risks, it may be reasonable, then, to look at the consequences of parental gonadal exposures. For a 1-rad parental gonadal dose, the same report estimates an increase of at most 0.0075% in the number of genetically effected live-born offspring. This increase should be compared against the average incidence of 6% to 10%. The risk of fetal gonadal exposure is, therefore, expected to be quite small, although not zero.

Blot and associates (1975) have studied the reproductive potential of children exposed *in utero* and have found no differences in frequency of childless marriages, number of births, or a difference in the interval between marriage and first birth.

The lack of data on this subject, either positive or negative, precludes any well-informed quantification of the risks. If there are genetic risks at diagnostic levels, they appear to be very small. It therefore seems prudent to use the cancer–malformation risks as decision criteria. Genetic risks, as we currently understand them, will not alter conclusions regarding medical management.

The possible effects of ionizing radiations on a conceptus are summarized in Table 4-2.

Ultrasound

There are no known deleterious effects to children exposed *in utero* to diagnostic ultrasound (Stratmeyer and Christman, 1982; Kremkau, 1982, 1983,

Table 4-2. Summary of Effects of Diagnostic Levels of Radiation (0–25 rad) on the Unborn[a,b]

Weeks Post-Conception	Gestation Stage	Effect				
		Prenatal Death	Small Head Size (SHS)	Severe Mental Retardation (SMR)	Other Malformation	Childhood Cancer
1st TRIMESTER 0— ... 2—	Preimplantation	Possible radiation-induced resorption	NDL	NDL	NDL	Higher risk period (see Table 4-1)
2— ... 6— 8—	Major organogenesis	NDL	Incidence of 1% per rad at Hiroshima, but causal nature of radiation is uncertain	NDL	Animal data suggest this is most sensitive stage, but NDL	
2nd & 3rd TRIMESTER 8— ... 15— 16—	Synaptogenesis Rapid neuron development and migration	NDL	NDL	SMR at 0.4% per rad from A-bomb, but radiation may not have been sole cause of this effect	NDL	Lesser risk period (see Table 4-1)
16— ... 38—			NDL	NDL		

[a]NDL = None established for humans at Diagnostic Levels.

[b]Effects from placental transfer of radionuclides are not included (see Chap. 1, section on "Radionuclide Examinations" and Chap. 4, section on "Other Forms

1984). Intensity levels for such devices are generally less than $200 \ mW/cm^2$ SPTA (Carson et al, 1978; Barnett and Kossoff, 1982; Nyborg, 1982). Several studies have reported negative results. Hellman and co-workers (1970) studied 1114 newborns of women who had apparently normal pregnancies and who received diagnostic ultrasound studies. Of these, 2.7% were born with abnormalities. The usual incidence of abnormalities at birth for similar groups is about 4%. The researchers concluded there was no observed increase in abnormalities resulting from diagnostic ultrasound examinations. This conclusion was independent of the gestation age when the examination was performed. As encouraging as these studies are, they do not strictly represent a scientifically controlled clinical study, and they therefore cannot be considered definitive.

Lyons (1982) studied 10,000 children who had received diagnostic ultrasound *in utero*. These were compared to 2000 children not exposed *in utero*. He also compared the *in utero* exposed children to 1000 unexposed control siblings. No differences in birth-defect rates or childhood-cancer rates were detected among the groups.

Scheidt and associates (1978) reported no statistically significant observation of increased birth defects, neurologic function deficits, or impaired growth for children exposed *in utero* to ultrasound and to amniocentesis. These were compared to two other groups of children; one that received only amniocentesis and the other that received neither. Grasp and neck reflexes were different among the groups, but these were normal by the time of discharge from the hospital.

David and co-workers (1975) reported an increase in fetal movement when exposing fetuses to continuous-wave ultrasound. This finding was challenged by Hertz and co-workers (1979), who found that, under similar circumstances, variations in fetal activity occur randomly and are not attributable to ultrasound.

Serr and associates (1971) reported an increase in chromosome breaks observed by amniocentesis after exposure to continuous-wave ultrasound. The results were not statistically significant, and several studies have subsequently reported no increase in chromosome aberrations from various tissues, including blood lymphocytes, amniotic fluid, cultured fibroblasts of aborted fetuses, or children 1 to 3 years after term (Abdulla et al, 1971; Falus et al, 1972; Watts and Stewart, 1972; Ikeuchi, 1973).

Testart and associates (1982) reported premature ovulation after ovarian ultrasonography. Based on this finding and speculation regarding possible adverse consequences, they recommend against ovarian ultrasonography in the days just before ovulation if the patient is trying to become pregnant.

Stark and associates (1984) studied 425 neonates previously exposed *in utero* to diagnostic ultrasound. The children were examined for a variety of possible adverse effects at birth and again when they were from 7 to 12 years of age. Results were compared against 381 matched controls. No biologically significant differences between the two groups were found. The exposed group did show a higher incidence of dyslexia, but the role of cultural and language biases may account for this difference. Further investigation is required to either support or disprove the causal nature of this finding.

The American Institute of Ultrasound in Medicine (AIUM) has reviewed many of these and other reports on biologic effects from ultrasound, including Dunn and Fry (1971), Wells (1974), Ulrich (1974), Reid and Sikov (1971), Hill (1972), Taylor (1974), Lele (1975), and the studies reviewed in Chapter 1. Based on this information, the AIUM has prepared the following statements (AIUM, 1977, 1983, 1984).

AIUM STATEMENT ON CLINICAL SAFETY

October 1982, revised March 1983 and October 1983

Diagnostic ultrasound has been in use for over 25 years. Given its known benefits and recognized efficacy for medical diagnosis, including use during human pregnancy, the American Institute of Ultrasound in Medicine herein addresses the clinical safety of such use:

No confirmed biologic effects on patients or instrument operators caused by exposure at intensities typical of present diagnostic ultrasound instruments have ever been reported. Although the possibility exists that such biologic effects may be identified in the future, current data indicate that the benefits to patients of the prudent use of diagnostic ultrasound outweigh the risks, if any, that may be present.

STATEMENT ON MAMMALIAN *IN VIVO* ULTRASONIC BIOLOGIC EFFECTS

August 1976, reaffirmed 1983

In the low-megahertz frequency range, there have been (as of this date) no independently confirmed significant biologic effects in mammalian tissues exposed to intensities* below 100 mW/cm^2. Furthermore, for ultrasonic exposure times[†] less than 500 seconds and greater than 1 second, such effects have not been demonstrated even at higher intensities, when the product of intensity* and exposure time[†] is less than 50 joules/cm^2.

Figure 4-4 graphically illustrates the combinations of intensity and exposure times that fall into this category. Also shown in Figure 4-4 is the upper limit of intensities from commercial obstetric devices. The current data suggest that it is highly unlikely that any deleterious effect will occur to a conceptus from the use of diagnostic ultrasound.

---

*Spatial peak temporal average (SPTA) as measured in a free field in water.
[†]Total time; this includes off-time as well as on-time for repeated pulse regimen.

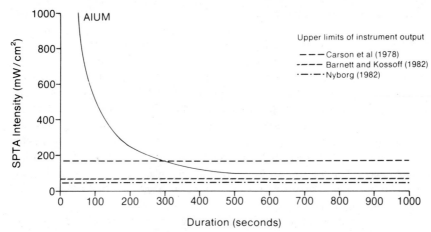

FIG. 4-4. Comparison of ultrasound instrument output with AIUM bioeffects statement. (Adapted from Kremkau FW: Biological effects and possible hazards. Clin Obstet Gynecol 10:395, 1983)

In view of the lack of evidence that ultrasound poses any risk to a mother or conceptus, Fletcher and Evans (1983) propose the use of ultrasound for early maternal–fetal bonding. This suggestion stirred several letters to the journal editor. Some affirmed the bonding effect (Bralow, 1983; Utian, 1983; Brick and Brick, 1983). The observation of a conceptus inside the womb can be exhilarating for the parents. One letter suggests it may have a beneficial psychological effect in that it heightens the awareness of the mother for good nutrition and proper care during pregnancy (Bralow, 1983). A few reports have supported this tenet (Milne and Rich, 1981; Kohn et al, 1980; Reading and Cox, 1982; Reading et al, 1982; Campbell et al, 1982). Another letter noted that, if an early fetus is discovered to be malformed, this knowledge may have a negative impact on the ability of the parents to cope with the pregnancy (Meier et al, 1983). Although knowledge regarding an untoward developmental status of an early pregnancy can be a benefit, the negative findings may have an adverse psychological effect that, theoretically, might lead to improper prenatal care on the part of the parents. In one letter it was noted that, based on an ultrasound study, a physician's fetus was erroneously diagnosed as dead (Feldman, 1983). Finally, another letter warned that although no deleterious effects have been demonstrated, this does not mean there are no risks (Bases et al, 1983). The letter's authors advise against the casual use of ultrasound. The use of ultrasound for early parental–fetal bonding remains controversial.

Magnetic Resonance

As of this writing, there is only meager evidence regarding the use of magnetic resonance (MR) during pregnancy. Smith and associates (1983, 1984) report on the use of MR in 15 first-trimester pregnancies. These studies focused on the potential for medical applications of MR in pregnant patients. All patients studied were previously scheduled for therapeutic abortion. They also report on one 32-week pregnancy referred for neurologic assessment of the mother. This patient delivered a normal child at birth. Foster and co-workers (1983) studied the prenatal imaging potential of MR using goats. This report did not address possible biologic effects. Sikov and associates (1979) found no increases in structural abnormalities in groups of mice exposed to 1 tesla *in utero.*

The information at this time is insufficient to make any substantial statements regarding the safety of this technique for conceptuses of pregnant women. The most encouraging results are those demonstrating no evidence that MR is mutagenic (see Chap. 1). However, further studies are necessary to establish its safety for use during pregnancy.

At this time, the Center for Devices and Radiological Health (1984) has placed this warning on all labels of devices approved by the Food and Drug Administration:

> The safety of the device when used to image fetuses and infants has not been established.

In the United Kingdom, the National Radiological Protection Board (1983) advises it might be prudent to exclude pregnant women in their first trimester from exposure to MR clinical imaging. These recommendations and warnings are subject to change as scientific studies on effects in pregnant animals become available.

References

Abdulla U, Dewhurst C, Campbell S et al: Effects of diagnostic ultrasound on maternal and fetal chromosomes. Lancet, 2:829, 1971

AIUM (American Institute of Ultrasound in Medicine): Statement on mammalian in-vivo ultrasonic biological effects. J Clin Ultrasound 5:3, 1977

AIUM (American Institute of Ultrasound in Medicine): AIUM bioeffects committee. J Ultrasound Med 2:R14, 1983

AIUM (American Institute of Ultrasound in Medicine): AIUM statement on clinical safety. J Ultrasound Med 3:R10, 1984

Barnett SB, Kossoff G: Ultrasonic exposure in static and real time echography. Ultrasound Med Biol 8:273, 1982

Bases R, Liebeskind D, Padawer J, Goodwin P: Letter: Maternal bonding in early fetal ultrasound examinations. N Engl J Med 309:115, 1983

BEIR (Committee on the Biological Effects of Ionizing Radiations): The Effects on Populations to Exposure to Low Levels of Ionizing Radiations: 1980. Washington, DC, National Academy Press, 1980

Blot WJ, Shimizu Y, Kato H et al: Frequency of marriage and live birth among survivors prenatally exposed to the atomic bomb. Am J Epidemiol 102:128, 1975

Bralow L: Letter: Maternal bonding in early fetal ultrasound examinations. N Engl J Med 309:114, 1983

Brent RL: Irradiation in pregnancy. In Sciarra JJ (ed): Davis' Gynecology and Obstetrics 2, p 1. New York, Harper and Row, 1972b

Brent RL: Radiations and other physical agents. In Wilson JG, Fraser FC (eds): Handbook of Teratology 1, p 1530 New York, Plenum Press, 1977

Brent RL: Teratology update: Radiation teratogenesis. Teratology 21:281, 1980

Brent RL: The effects of embryonic and fetal exposure to x-ray, microwaves, and ultrasound. Clin Obstet Gynecol (2)26:484, 1983

Brent RL, Gorson RO: Radiation exposure in pregnancy. Curr Probl Radiol 2:1, 1972a

Brick J, Brick J: Letter: Maternal bonding in early fetal ultrasound examinations. N Engl J Med 309:116, 1983

Campbell S, Reading AE, Cox DN et al: Ultrasound scanning in pregnancy: The short term psychological effects of early real-time scans. J Psychosomatic Ob Gyn 1:57, 1982

Carson PL, Fischella PR, Oughton TV: Ultrasonic power and intensities produced by diagnostic ultrasound equipment. Ultrasound Med Biol 3:341, 1978

Center for Devices and Radiological Health, Office of Device Evaluation, 8757 Georgia Avenue, Silver Spring, Maryland, 20970, Personal communication, 1984

Choi NW, Klaponski FA: On neural-tube defects: An epidemiological elicitation of etiological factors. Neurology 20:399, 1970

Court-Brown WM, Doll R, Hill AB: Incidence of leukaemia after exposure to diagnostic radiation *in utero*. Br Med J 2:1539, 1960

David H, Weaver JB, Pearson JF: Doppler ultrasound and fetal activity. Br Med J 3:62, 1975

Diamond EL, Schmerler H, Lilienfeld AM: The relationship of intrauterine radiation to subsequent mortality and development of leukemia in children. Am J Epidemiol 97:283, 1973

Dobbing J, Sands J: Quantitative growth and development of human brain. Arch Dis Child 48:757, 1973

Dunn F, Fry FJ: Ultrasonic threshold dosages for the mammalian central nervous system. IEEE Trans Biomed Eng BME-18:253, 1971

Edmonds DK, Lindsay KS, Miller JF et al: Early embryonic mortality in women. Fertil Steril 38:447, 1982

Falus M, Korany G, Sobel M et al: Follow-up studies on infants examined by ultrasound during fetal age. Orv Hetil 113:2119, 1972

Feldman V: Letter: Maternal bonding in early fetal ultrasound examinations. N Engl J Med 309:115, 1983

Fletcher JC, Evans MI: Maternal bonding in early fetal ultrasound examinations. N Engl J Med 308:392, 1983

Foster MA, Knight CH, Rimmington JE et al: Fetal imaging by nuclear magnetic resonance: A study in goats. Radiology 149:193, 1983

Graham S et al: Preconception, intrauterine and postnatal irradiation as related leukemia. Natl Cancer Inst Monogr 19:347, 1966

Granroth G: Defects of the central nervous system in Finland IV. Associations with diagnostic x-ray examinations. Am J Obstet Gynecol 133:191, 1979

Hammer-Jacobsen E: Therapeutic abortion on account of x-ray examination during pregnancy. Dan Med Bull 6:113, 1959

Heinonen OP, Slone D, Shapiro S: Birth Defects and Drugs in Pregnancy. p 516, Littleton, Massachusettes, Publishing Sciences Group, 1977

Hellman LM, Duffus GM, Donald I et al: Safety of diagnostic ultrasound in obstetrics. Lancet p 1133, 1970

Hertz RH, Timor-Tritsch I, Dierker LJ et al: Continuous ultrasound and fetal movement. Am J Obstet Gynecol 135:152, 1979

Hill CR: Ultrasonic exposure thresholds for changes in cells and tissues. J Acoust Soc Am 52:667, 1972

Hoffman DA, Felten RP, Cyr WH: Effects of Ionizing Radiation on the Developing Embryo and Fetus, HHS publication (FDA) 81-8170. Rockville, Maryland, Bureau of Radiological Health, 1981

Ikeuchi T, Sasaki M, Oshimuoa M et al: Ultrasound and embryonic chromosomes. Br Med J p 112, 1973

Jablon S, Kato H: Childhood cancer in relation to prenatal exposure to atomic bomb radiation. Lancet, p 1000, 1970

Jacobsen L, Mellemgaard L: Anomalies of the eyes in descendants of woman irradiated with small x-ray dose during age of fertility. Acta Ophthalmol 46:352, 1968

Kerr GD, Pace JV, Scott WH: Tissue kerma versus distance relationships for initial nuclear radiation from the atomic bombs at Hiroshima and Nagasaki. US–Japan Joint Workshop for Reassessment of Atomic Bomb Radiation Dosimetry in Hiroshima and Nagasaki, pp 57–98. Hiroshima, Radiation Effects Research Foundation, 1983

Kinlen LJ, Acheson ED: Diagnostic irradiation, congenital malformations and spontaneous abortion. Br J Radiol 41:648, 1968

Kneale GW, Stewart AM: Mantel-Haenszel analysis of Oxford data. I. Independent effects of several birth factors including fetal irradiation. J Natl Cancer Inst 56:879, 1976a

Kneale GW, Stewart AM: Mantel-Haenszel analysis of Oxford data. II. Independent effects of fetal irradiation subfactors. J Natl Cancer Inst 57:1009, 1976b

Kohn CL, Nelson A, Weiner S: Gravidas responses to realtime ultrasound fetal image. J Obstet/Gynecol Nurs, March/April, 1980

Kremkau FW: How safe is obstetric ultrasound? Contemporary Ob Gyn 20:182, 1982

Kremkau FW: Biological effects and possible hazards. Clin Obstet Gynecol 10:395, 1983

Kremkau FW: Safety and long-term effects of ultrasound: What to tell your patients. Clin Obstet Gynecol 27:269, 1984

Lele PP: Ultrasonic teratology in mouse and man, Excerpta Medica International Congress Series No. 363, Proceedings of the Second European Congress on Ultrasonics in Medicine, p 22 1975

Lyons EA: In: Fetal ultrasound: How safe? Sci News 121:396, 1982

MacMahon B: Prenatal x-ray exposure and childhood cancer. J Natl Cancer Inst 28:1173, 1962

Meier PR, Good W, Clewell WH et al: Maternal bonding in early fetal ultrasound examinations. N Engl J Med 309:114, 1983

Miller RW, Blot NJ: Small head size after *in-utero* exposure to atomic radiation. Lancet 2:784, 1972

Miller RW, Mulvihill JJ: Small head size after atomic irradiation. Teratology 14:355, 1976

Miller JF, Williamson E, Glue J et al: Fetal loss following implantation: A prospective study. Lancet 1:554, 1980

Milne LS, Rich OJ: Cognitive and affective aspects of the responses of pregnant women to sonography. Matern Child Nurs 10:15, 1981

Mole RH: Consequences of pre-natal radiation exposure for post-natal development — A review. Int J Radiat Biol 42:1, 1982

Monson RR, MacMahon B: Prenatal x-ray exposure and cancer in children. In Boice JD, Fraumeni JF (eds): Radiation Carcinogenesis: Epidemiology and Biological Significance, pp 97–105. New York, Raven Press, 1984

National Radiological Protection Board: Revised guidance on acceptable limits of exposure during nuclear magnetic clinical imaging. Br J Radiol 56:974, 1983

Nokkentved K: Effect of Diagnostic Radiation upon the Human Fetus, p 228. Copenhagen, Munksgaard, 1968

Nyborg WL: Ultrasonic intensities generated by real-time devices. In Winsberg F, Cooperburg PL (eds): Clinics in Diagnostic Ultrasound. Real-Time Ultrasonography, vol 10, p 15. New York, Churchill Livingstone, 1982

Otake M, Schull WJ: *In utero* exposure to A-bomb radiation and mental retardation: A reassessment. Br J Radiol 57:409, 1984

Reading AE, Cox DN: The effects of ultrasound examination on maternal anxiety levels. J Behav Med 5:237, 1982

Reading AE, Campbell S, Cox D et al: Health beliefs and health care behavior in pregnancy. Psychol Med 12:379, 1982

Reid JM, Sikov MR (eds): Interaction of Ultrasound and Biological Tissues, HEW publication (FDA), 78-8008. Rockville, Maryland, Bureau of Radiological Health, 1971

Rugh R: X-irradiation effects on the human fetus. J Pediat 52:531, 1958

Scheidt PC, Stanley F, Bryla DA: One-year follow-up of infants exposed to ultrasound *in utero.* Am J Obstet Gynecol 131:743, 1978

Serr DM, Padeh B, Zakett H et al: Studies on the effects of ultrasonic waves on the fetus. In Huntingford PJ, Beard RW, Hytten et al (eds): Proceedings of the Second European Congress in Perinatal Medicine, London, 1971. New York, Karger, 1971

Sikov MR, Mahlum DD, Montgomery LD et al: Development of mice after intrauterine exposure to direct current magnetic fields. Biological Effects of Extremely Low Frequency Electro-Magnetic Fields: Proceedings of the 18th Hanford Life Sciences Symposium, Richland, Washington, 1978, pp 462–473. Springfield, VA, Technical Information Center, US Department of Energy, 1979

Smith FW, Adam AH, Phillips WDP: NMR imaging in pregnancy. Lancet 1/8:61, January 1983

Smith FW, MacLennan F, Abramovich DR et al: NMR imaging in human pregnancy: A preliminary study. Magnetic Resonance Imaging 2:57, 1984

Stark CR, Orleans M, Haverkamp AD et al: Short- and long-term risks after exposure to diagnostic ultrasound. Obstet Gynecol 63:194, 1984

Sternberg J: Radiation risk in pregnancy. Clin Obstet Gynecol 16 (1):235, 1973

Stewart AM, Kneale GW: Radiation dose effects in relation to obstetric x-rays and childhood cancers. Lancet, p 1185, June 1970

Stoffer SS, Hamburger JI: Inadvertent ^{131}I therapy for hypothyroidism in the first trimester of pregnancy. J Nucl Med 17:146, 1976

Stratmeyer ME, Christman CL: Biological effects of ultrasound. Women Health 7:65, 1982

Tabuchi A: Fetal disorder due to ionizing radiation. Hiroshima J Med Sci 13:125, 1964

Tabuchi A, Nakagawa S, Hirai T et al: Fetal hazards due to x-ray diagnosis during pregnancy. Hiroshima J Med Sci 16:49, 1967

Taylor KJW: Current status of toxicity investigations. J Clin Ultrasound 2:149, 1974

Testart J, Thebault A, Frydman R: Premature ovulation after ovarian ultrasonography. Br J Obstet Gynaecol 89:694, 1982

Ulrich WD: Ultrasound Dosage for Experimental Use on Human Beings. Report of the Naval Medical Research Institute, Project M4306. 01-1010BSK9, 19 August 1971 (See also IEEE Trans Biomed Eng BME-21, p 48, 1974)

UNSCEAR (United Nations Scientific Committee on the Effects of Atomic Radiation): Biological Effects of Irradiation *In Utero,* 1984 (in press)

Utian WH: Maternal bonding in early fetal ultrasound examinations. N Engl J Med 309:115, 1983

Villumsen AL: Environmental Factors in Congenital Malformations, pp 130–142. Copenhagen, FADL's Forlag, 1970

Watts P, Stewart C: The effect of fetal heart monitoring by ultrasound on maternal and fetal chromosomes. J Obstet Gynaecol Br Commonw 79:715, 1972

Wells PNT: The possibility of harmful biological effects in ultrasonic diagnosis. In Reneman RS (ed): Proceedings of the Symposium on Cardiovascular Applications of Ultrasound, p 1. New York, American Elsevier, 1974

Wood JW, Keehn RJ, Kawamoto S et al: The growth and development of children exposed *in utero* to the atomic bombs in Hiroshima and Nagasaki. Am J Public Health 57:1374, 1967

Yamazaki JN: A review of the literature on the radiation dosage required to cause manifest central nervous system disturbances from *in utero* and postnatal exposure. Pediatrics 37:877, 1966

Note Added in Proof

An article entitled "Prenatal X-ray exposure and childhood cancer in twins," by Harvey, Boice, Honeyman, and Flannery, was published in the *New England Journal of Medicine* 5:541, 1985. The data presented in that paper are consistent with the data presented in this book and do not alter any of the conclusions drawn in this text.

Part II
The Clinical Management
of the Pregnant Patient
Needing Diagnostic Study

PreExamination Flowchart

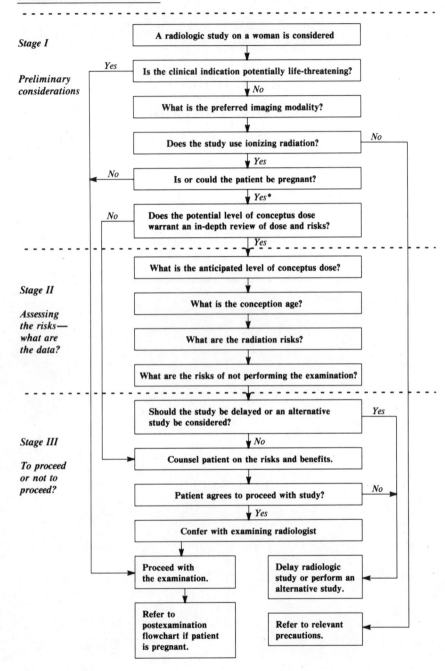

Stage I

Preliminary considerations

A radiologic study on a woman is considered

Yes — Is the clinical indication potentially life-threatening?

No — What is the preferred imaging modality?

Does the study use ionizing radiation? — No

Yes

No — Is or could the patient be pregnant?

Yes*

No — Does the potential level of conceptus dose warrant an in-depth review of dose and risks?

Yes

Stage II

Assessing the risks— what are the data?

What is the anticipated level of conceptus dose?

What is the conception age?

What are the radiation risks?

What are the risks of not performing the examination?

Stage III

To proceed or not to proceed?

Should the study be delayed or an alternative study be considered? — Yes

No

Counsel patient on the risks and benefits.

Patient agrees to proceed with study? — No

Yes

Confer with examining radiologist

Proceed with the examination.

Delay radiologic study or perform an alternative study.

Refer to postexamination flowchart if patient is pregnant.

Refer to relevant precautions.

*Studies not medically warranted should be delayed until after term.

80

Chapter 5
Stage I,
Preliminary Considerations

```
┌─────────────────────────────────────────┐
│ A radiologic study on a woman is          │
│ considered                                │
└─────────────────────────────────────────┘
                    │
                    ▼
┌─────────────────────────────────────────┐
│ Is the clinical indication potentially    │
│ life-threatening?                         │
└─────────────────────────────────────────┘
```

When a woman requires an emergency radiologic examination, there should be no hesitation to do the study. If the patient is able to communicate or if a relative or friend is readily accessible, a brief inquiry to determine whether the patient is known to be pregnant is useful. First, the answer may explain some findings of preliminary tests and physical examination. Second, if she is indeed pregnant, the radiologist will be alerted to the fact and will avoid inadvertent radiation exposure to the conceptus. If the study requires direct exposure to the conceptus and there are no satisfactory diagnostic alternatives, the radiologist should proceed and not hesitate to properly complete the examination.

For elective procedures, the question of whether a patient requires a radiologic study is usually addressed early in the workup. It is based on an evaluation of the symptoms, history, physical examination, and, sometimes, laboratory data. Nonphysicians often think this is a simple yes or no decision. In fact, judgment and experience concerning the importance and significance of positive or negative findings and the influence of this information on patient care are all involved. In a basic sense, the physician makes a determination of benefit and risk each time a radiographic examination is contemplated. The physician also weighs the fact that there is a benefit–risk decision to be made in regard to not performing the examination. (Factors such as cost versus benefit may additionally influence the decision to obtain the examination.)

Prior to requesting an elective radiologic study for a woman, a few preliminary questions should be addressed. The following is the first of these.

What is the preferred imaging modality?

The range of radiologic examinations has increased dramatically in recent years. A variety of studies using ionizing radiations provide greater or lesser quantities of information. Certain studies may require more or less radiation exposure. The idea that information and radiation dosage are directly related is simplistic. For example, a fluoroscopic study of the abdomen may deliver more radiation to the patient than a carefully planned computed tomographic (CT) study.

More important, the array of effective imaging studies now includes magnetic resonance (MR) and ultrasound, frequently providing detailed information without exposing the patient to ionizing radiation. MR imaging for general diagnosis as well as for examination of the conceptus is currently undergoing clinical evaluation (Smith et al, 1984, 1983; Foster et al, 1983). Ultrasonography is used to diagnose many conditions that previously required ionizing radiation. These include nephrolithiasis, cholelithiasis, cysts (ovarian, pancreatic), renal pathologies (polycystic kidneys, renal atrophy), and medicosurgical conditions (pancreatitis, retrocecal appendicitis, ectopic pregnancy, missing intrauterine contraceptive device).

Sonography can periodically monitor the progress of the aforementioned conditions to see if surgical intervention is necessary. It should be used in conjunction with other laboratory tests and sound clinical judgment.

Ultrasonography has replaced ionizing radiologic imaging for some procedures used in management of high-risk pregnancy. This includes its use in genetic amniocentesis, intrauterine fetal transfusion, placental localization, and determination of fetal lie and position. Many fetal anomalies such as anencephaly, hydrocephaly, spina bifida, and cystic hygroma may be ruled out using ultrasound. Multiple pregnancies and amniotic fluid abnormalities (oligohydramnios, polyhydramnios) can also be easily detected.

The technological and diagnostic capabilities of imaging procedures are continually expanding. It is difficult for referring physicians to remain abreast of the most contemporary equipment and techniques. For this reason, it is recommended that they consult with a radiologist regarding the patient's diagnostic evaluation. The radiologist may be able to recommend examinations that avoid ionizing radiation or alternative examinations that use less ionizing radiation. This is particularly important because of the rapid advances in MR imaging.

Does the study use ionizing radiation?

All x-ray and nuclear radiologic studies involve ionizing radiation. Ultrasound and MR are nonionizing imaging techniques. There have been no reports of ill effects resulting from obstetric ultrasound, but it may not be totally innocuous (see Chap. 4). The potential consequences of a MR study on a pregnant woman have not been rigorously researched. The currently used MR imaging techniques produce no known biologic damage. More research is necessary to determine whether there are risks associated with this technology.

If the study requested does not involve ionizing radiation, we advise the referring physician to consult with the examining radiologist for any precautions and preparations that may be relevant to that modality. Because MR imaging involves the use of very strong magnetic fields, patients who have surgical clips or other implanted metal devices may be susceptible to internal injury.

For ultrasound, the patient should be properly prepared (*e.g.*, the bladder should be full for uterine study). The only precaution is that the examining personnel limit the duration of the study to the time required to obtain the necessary information. Even though we know of no risk relevant to diagnostic ultrasound, it is clear that limiting the duration of the study will minimize any potential risk that may exist.

A National Institutes of Health Consensus Development Conference (1983) on the use of diagnostic ultrasound recommends the following guidelines for the use of ultrasound in obstetrics:

- Ultrasound examination in pregnancy should be performed for a specific medical indication.
- Data on clinical efficacy and safety do not allow a recommendation for routine screening at this time.
- Ultrasound examinations performed solely to satisfy the family's desire to know the fetal sex, to view the fetus, or to obtain a picture of the fetus should be discouraged.

- Visualization of the fetus solely for educational or commercial demonstrations without medical benefit to the patient should not be performed.
- Prior to an ultrasound examination, patients should be informed of the clinical indication for ultrasound, specific benefit, potential risk, and alternatives, if any.
- The patient should be supplied with information about the exposure time and intensity, if requested.
- Given that the full potential of diagnostic ultrasound is critically dependent on examiner training and experience, minimum training requirements and the uniform credentialing for all physicians and sonographers performing ultrasound examinations is recommended.
- All health-care providers who use this modality should demonstrate adequate knowledge of the basic principles of ultrasound, equipment, record keeping requirements, indications, and safety.
- All settings in which these examinations are conducted should assure the patient's dignity and privacy.

If the examination to be requested involves the use of ionizing radiation, the following question should be asked next.

Is or could the patient be pregnant?

ACTIONS PRIOR TO REFERRAL FOR RADIOLOGIC STUDY

Menstrual history is the most important step in ascertaining reproductive status. It is customary for referring physicians to acquire a brief menstrual history of all female patients as part of their routine medical care. It should include age of menarche, regularity and duration of menstrual cycles, and the date and duration of the last normal menstrual period.

For many radiographic studies, menstrual history is sufficient to determine if the patient is, may be, or is not pregnant. Conventional radiography of the extremities, head, and thorax, and computed or conventional tomography of the head deliver minimal amounts of radiation to the uterus, and any medical benefit from them outweighs the surmised risks should the patient be pregnant. Information about a late menstruation is useful to the radiologist prior to these examinations because it calls attention to the need for careful radiographic positioning of the patient in the event that she is pregnant (see next section of flowchart).

The reproductive status of a woman should be more thoroughly investigated prior to referral for abdominal or pelvic radiography, special procedures, CT of the chest or abdomen, or nuclear medicine studies. A significant shift to an earlier menarche and a later menopause has extended the childbearing period of women in the United States. It is not uncommon for adolescent or premenopausal women to conceive. Reproductive status should be considered for all women between the ages of puberty ($\sim$12 years) and menopause ($\sim$50 years). The referring physician should solicit a contraceptive and sexual history from the patient when appropriate. Careful attention should be given to the patient's compliance with contraceptive methods. In women who are reluctant to reveal information relevant to a possible pregnancy, a sympathetic, nonjudgmental counseling session regarding the need for the sexual history and information pertinent to possible pregnancy should be held.

Symptoms suggestive of pregnancy should be followed up with a pregnancy test. Quantitative analysis of the beta subunit of human chorionic gonadotropins (HCG) in serum is specific for pregnancy. A urine pregnancy test is not nearly as sensitive or specific even if radioimmunoassay is used. The serum test may be positive as early as 7 days after the first missed period. It has also been found positive even before implantation in some women. If the test results disagree with clinical findings, a possibility is ectopic pregnancy. The HCG titer in this condition will cease to increase, in contrast to normal pregnancy where it doubles every 24 to 48 hours.

Pelvic examination can confirm pregnancy around 8 to 10 weeks menstrual age (6 to 8 weeks conception age). However, retroflextion of the uterus may cause difficulty in diagnosing pregnancy by this method.

ACTIONS BY THE RADIOLOGIST

Posters (Fig. 5-1) that ask the patient to inform the radiologist about a possible pregnancy are helpful in screening ambulatory patients at the radiology department. Such posters are often not seen by nonambulatory patients who are escorted to the examination suites.

Some radiologists instruct their technologists to ask all female patients (or appropriate guardians of adolescents) between the ages of 12 and 50 about possible pregnancy before they have an abdominal or pelvic radiographic examination. A box on the examination request form is checked when this has been done. Other radiologists prefer that the patient complete a questionnaire. This has the advantage of avoiding potentially embarrassing confrontations for adolescents and other patients. Two questions are appropriate: (1) Could you be pregnant? and (2) What was the date of onset of your last menstrual period? A yes answer to the first question is brought to the attention of the radiologist, who can acquire a more complete reproductive history. In regard to the second question, some radiologists more thoroughly review the question of pregnancy only if the onset of last menses exceeds 4 weeks. This is because there is no known risk of malformation if the patient is less than 2 weeks pregnant. However, there

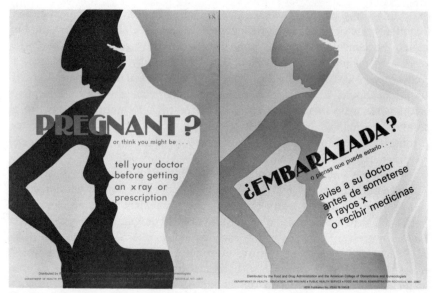

FIG. 5-1.   Posters useful in screening pregnant patients before radiologic examination.

may be a small risk of radiation-induced childhood cancer (see Table 4-1). For this reason, others prefer to more thoroughly investigate possible pregnancy if the onset exceeds 10 days. This is consistent with the "10-day rule" (see Chap. 7). If pregnancy is not ruled out, the radiologist consults with the referring physician to decide if a pregnancy test is indicated. This depends on the urgency of the study, the gestation age, and whether or not the patient's symptoms are perhaps due to pregnancy. (These issues are discussed in more detail later.)

BENEFITS OF INVESTIGATING PREGNANCY STATUS

In light of public awareness that radiation can cause health problems, pregnant women and their families are highly sensitive to issues surrounding exposure of unborn children to radiation. This inquiry regarding pregnancy has several possible beneficial effects:

1. *The patient's complaint may be due to pregnancy.* In this case, both the patient and the conceptus would be spared unnecessary radiation. The clinician must be aware of the symptoms of pregnancy that may mimic other conditions. These include nausea, vomiting, dizziness, headache, and shortness of breath. Confusion with medicosurgical conditions may also arise from round-ligament spasm (*e.g.,* appendicitis).

An example is the older obese patient who presents with symptoms of cholelithiasis. Pregnancy is not always considered before the patient is referred for an oral cholecystogram. When that study proves negative, a barium enema examination is sometimes ordered. Only afterward is it learned that the patient is pregnant. In some actual cases conceptuses received between 2 and 10 rad of radiation. The conceptus doses in these obese patients can be considerably larger than those for thinner patients.

Another case that sometimes occurs is that of the young unmarried patient who presents with abdominal pain and denies any possibility of pregnancy. These patients frequently undergo similar radiographic evaluation before pregnancy is diagnosed. A serum beta-HCG pregnancy test prior to referral for radiographic study may sometimes be appropriate.

2. The patient is made aware of the physician's efforts to consider the issue. If she might be or is pregnant, her questions can be answered, and she then has the opportunity to consider the advice and counsel of the physician before proceeding with the study. In the case where the study is urgently needed, she will be less likely to be upset if pregnancy is confirmed afterward.

3. The onset of the last menses may have occurred within a time period not exceeding her normal menstrual cycle. In this situation the patient is either not pregnant or is presumably not more than 2 weeks pregnant. The suspected risks from diagnostic radiation delivered at this time are induced resorbtion or possible childhood cancer. There are no suspected risks from malformation (see Table 4-2). The physician may want to proceed with the study at this time to avoid the risk of small head size and mental retardation should the study become imperative weeks later. Special circumstances exist for studies involving long-lived radionuclides (see Chap. 7).

4. If the patient is not pregnant, a note to the radiologist stating this will forego unnecessary delays in the examination since the radiologist will then know that there is no need to address the issue.

5. If the patient is pregnant
   a) The referring physician or the radiologist may be able to suggest an alternative study that either requires less or no ionizing radiation.
   b) There are certain studies, performed for nonsymptomatic reasons (*e.g.,* preemployment physical examinations, research applications), that can be delayed beyond term.
   c) It may be possible to delay the study until a time beyond the 15th week if the conceptus is at an age sensitive to radiation-induced small head size (weeks 2 to 15) or severe mental retardation (weeks 8 to 15). This would also reduce hypothesized cancer risk. However, delaying the study because of a very early pregnancy may be counterproductive if the patient's condition should worsen and the study be-

come imperative during weeks 8 to 15, when the conceptus is at risk for severe mental retardation.

d) Precautions in performing the study can be taken to ensure that radiation exposure to the conceptus is kept as low as possible.

ACTION WHEN THE PATIENT IS NOT PREGNANT

If the patient is not pregnant, some authorities advise that she be counseled not to become pregnant for at least 2 months after the study (NCRP, 1971, 1977). The basis for this is a study in mice that indicates that such an interval is effective in reducing radiation-induced mutations (Russell, 1965). Although this advice would conceivably eliminate the remote possibility of some genetically induced defects, the likelihood that such events might occur at diagnostic levels is very small. This advice may be reasonable only for patients who receive large doses of radiation (exceeding 25 rad) to the gonads. Indeed, although the NCRP (1977) advises

> In cases where pregnancy is not suspected, the patient should be advised that she should not run the risk of pregnancy until two months after the examination of the abdomen or pelvis has been performed.

In Report No. 39 the NCRP (1971) specifies at what doses this is necessary:

> Nevertheless it may be advisable for patients receiving high doses to the gonads (over 25 rads) to wait *several* months after such exposure before conceiving additional offspring.

If pregnancy is confirmed or is a possibility, then we ask the following.

Does the potential level of conceptus dose warrant an in-depth review of dose and risks?

Radiologic examinations of the extremities (excluding the upper femur), thorax, and head (including dental x rays and computed and conventional tomography) deliver very small amounts of radiation to the conceptus (see Table 3-1). The dose from many of these studies is usually a small fraction of the amount of naturally occurring radiation that the conceptus will receive during the 9 months of gestation. This natural environmental radiation is around 50 mrem to 100 mrem to the conceptus per gestation, depending on where one lives. When these radiologic studies are performed properly (*e.g.,* proper collimation and shielding of the uterus by a lead apron) the dose to the conceptus is often less than 10 mrem. To lend some perspective to this dose level, an unborn child of a woman living in Denver receives about a 50-mrem greater dose during gestation from background radiation than does the unborn child of a woman living in Miami. The risks associated with these doses and the lower doses from the aforementioned radiologic examinations are very small. The radiologic dose to the conceptus does not warrant a thorough investigation. The patient should be counseled that the risk is minimal.

A modest extra effort can guarantee that the dose to the conceptus is as small as possible. The status of the patient (not pregnant, possibly pregnant, or pregnant) should be communicated to the radiologist. If the patient is pregnant or might be pregnant, this calls attention to the need for particular care in establishing radiographic technique. The personnel performing this study should make sure that the patient is positioned in such a way that her pelvis does not accidentally intercept the radiation field. Her pelvis can be shielded with a lead apron to ensure that radiation exposure is kept to the barest minimum. The patient should be advised that this precaution is taken, not because there is a significant threat to the conceptus, but simply to guarantee that the dose to the conceptus is kept well below the natural environmental levels of radiation. It is the responsibility of radiologists to ensure that their personnel are properly trained so that appropriate care is afforded their patients.

Some extra-abdominal studies may deliver more radiation to the conceptus than the minimal amounts previously discussed. These include cerebral angiography, conventional tomography of the chest, cardiac catheterization, and CT of the chest. None of these studies is likely to deliver more than 1 rad to the conceptus unless the studies are repeated or there is direct exposure of the conceptus (*e.g.,* pelvic fluoroscopy performed for placement of a catheter) or, as in the case of CT, a decision is made to perform abdominal CT while the patient is on the table. The NCRP (1977) states that "At dose levels below one rad, the probability of detectable effect induced by such exposures is so small as to be outweighed by any significant medical benefits." As long as precautions are taken to avoid direct exposure of the abdomen during these examinations, the dose to the uterus is not expected to exceed 1 rad. However, we previously recommended that a possibility of pregnancy should be followed through with a pregnancy test prior to referral for these studies. This is important in order to alert the radiologists of this fact so that they are aware of the pregnancy and avoid inadvertent and unnecessary exposures to the conceptus. For example, consider the case where a patient undergoes thoracic CT, and the radiologic findings suggest that an abdominal series is appropriate. The radiologist may wish to proceed with the abdominal study while the patient is there. Dose-limiting options will be initiated only if the radiologist knows of the pregnancy. The options are to proceed as planned, to do the study using less radiation than conventionally used, to do the study on a better machine, to avoid scanning the uterus, to cancel the study, or to do a different study.

If the study requested is a special-procedure examination that requires brief abdominal exposure for placement of a catheter, knowledge of the pregnancy will help the radiologist in limiting the dose to the conceptus. For example, cerebral arteriography is a lengthy procedure that requires multiple radiographs of the head and fluoroscopy of the thorax and possibly the pelvis for placement of the catheter. Irradiation of the conceptus from the cranial radiographs themselves is very small. Gray and associates (1981) report that, for radiographs in the head region, the dose to the uterus is only a few tenths of a millirad per roentgen entrance exposure. For 60 appropriately coned head arteriograms, the conceptus dose is probably less than 10 mrad. The contribution of radiation from thoracic fluoroscopy during placement of the catheter is small as long as the fluoroscopy is confined to the area of the chest. A quantification of this level of radiation is not possible in the general case since it will depend on the duration of the study, and the equipment and techniques used by the physician. Ten minutes of fluoroscopy confined to the chest is not likely to result in more than 0.5 rad to the conceptus. If a catheter is inserted through a femoral artery, there will be fluoroscopy in the region of the pelvis. This elevates the dose to the uterus. It would be unusual for doses from this fluoroscopy to exceed 1 or 2 rad because of the short duration of the exposure. Knowledge of the pregnancy would alert the neuroradiologist to the need for keeping exposures to the pelvic area brief.

CONCLUSIONS

Extra-abdominal radiographic studies, including special procedures, are not likely to exceed a 1-rad dose to the conceptus if the radiologist is aware of the pregnancy. In this case, a conscientious effort can be made to minimize direct irradiation of the conceptus. A more thorough investigation of dose and risk would not normally be required unless multiple special-procedure studies are anticipated or an abdominal study is subsequently performed.

For abdominal radiographic examinations and studies involving radionuclides, it is reasonable to more thoroughly review the dose levels and the radiation risks. These are discussed in the next chapter.

REFERENCES

National Institutes of Health Consensus Panel: Tentative Consensus Statement on the Use of Diagnostic Ultrasound Imaging in Pregnancy, Washington, DC, December 12, 1983

Foster MA, Knight CH, Rimmington JE et al: Fetal imaging by nuclear magnetic resonance: A study in goats. Radiology 149:193, 1983

Gray JE, Ragozzino MW, Van Lysel MS et al: Normalized organ doses for various diagnostic radiologic procedures. Am J Radiol 137:463, 1981

NCRP (National Council on Radiation Protection and Measurements): Basic Radiation Protection Criteria, NCRP Report No. 39. Washington, DC, National Council on Radiation Protection and Measurements, 1971

NCRP (National Council on Radiation Protection and Measurements): Medical Radiation Exposure of Pregnant and Potentially Pregnant Women, NCRP Report No. 54. Washington, DC, National Council on Radiation Protection and Measurements, 1977

Russell WL: Effect of the interval between irradiation and conception on mutation frequency in female mice. Proc Nat Acad Sci 54:1552, 1965

Smith FW, Adam AH, Phillips WDP: NMR imaging in pregnancy. Lancet 1:61, 1983

Smith FW, MacLennan F, Abramovich DR et al: NMR imaging in human pregnancy: A preliminary study. Magnetic Resonance Imaging 2:57, 1984

Chapter 6
Stage II,
Assessing the Risks—
What Are the Data?

Before any risk evaluation can be made, it is first necessary to answer the following question.

> ## What is the anticipated conceptus dose?

Abdominal examinations and radionuclide studies are of particular concern either because of the extent of the examination, the proximity of the x-ray beam to the uterus, or the distribution of radioactivity in the patient. These examinations may reasonably be suspected to contribute levels of radiation to the uterus that might significantly exceed the minimal radiation levels of previously discussed extra-abdominal examinations.

For upper abdominal radiographic examinations the dose to the conceptus can be on the order of a few rad, but is usually much less. Radiation dose as a function of distance from the edge of primary x-ray beam is approximated in Figure A-10. These data indicate that only a very small fraction of the x rays from upper abdominal examinations need reach the uterus if care is taken to confine the x-ray beam to the necessary anatomy. Surveys indicate that radiographic filming during upper abdominal examinations (*e.g.*, upper GI series, cholecystography) has delivered doses anywhere from 5 mrad to 1600 mrad to the conceptus (see Table 3-4). This does not include the additional dose from fluoroscopy. Using contemporary imaging equipment, proper collimation, and good technique, it would be unusual for uterine doses (including those from fluoroscopy) to exceed 2 rad if the examination is confined to the upper abdomen.

Radiographic filming for examinations of the lower abdomen can deliver considerably higher doses to the uterus. The survey data listed in Table 3-4 show that doses to the uterus from barium enema radiography have ranged from 28 mrad to about 12,600 mrad, with an average uterine dose of about 1,200 mrad. In addition, a typical dose from fluoroscopy of the lower abdomen might be 1 rad to 3 rad. The dose can be substantially less or substantially more, depending on factors discussed in Chapter 3. For the lowest dose cases, the increased risk is minimal. The highest doses are unusual. Such doses may be delivered during detailed studies of the sigmoid colon, in obese women, or by suboptimal imaging equipment.

For studies that directly expose the lower abdomen, a radiological physicist can approximate the dose to the uterus. To do so, the physicist requires information on patient size, and the radiographic techniques and equipment to be used. Direct consultation with the radiologist who will perform the study can provide some estimate as to the number of radiographic films required and the anticipated duration of the fluoroscopic examination. Dose-estimation techniques are reviewed in Appendix A.

For abdominal computed tomography (CT), if the uterus *is not* in the view of the x-ray beam, conceptus dose should not exceed 3 rad for a single series of routine scans. In the usual case, the dose is not likely to exceed 1 rad. If the uterus *is* in direct view, conceptus dose will be greater. In some exceptional cases, when special CT procedures are used, the dose can be substantially higher (more than 10 rad). The anticipated dose can be estimated by a radiological physicist.

Doses from nuclear radiologic studies are more difficult to estimate accurately. The reasons for this are discussed in Chapter 3. These include uncertainties regarding the metabolism of the radionuclide as well as variations in patient size and the distances of maternal organs from the uterus. Conceptus dose from radioactivity in the bladder can only be approximated if the radionuclide is eliminated through the urinary tract. Assumptions have to be made regarding the periodicity of voiding. Placental transfer of the radionuclide can substantially increase dose to the organs of the conceptus. The amount of transfer is not usually well known. Table 3-5 lists some expected doses to the conceptus per millicurie of radiopharmaceutical administered to the mother. The limitations of these estimates are specified in the table. These probably represent the best guidance regarding conceptus dose from radiopharmaceutical studies. However, it must be remembered that these are only estimates that may be substantially in error (by a factor of 2 or more if the radiation does not cross the placenta, and by considerably larger amounts if possible placental uptake and transfer is not adequately accounted for in the calculation).

For radionuclides not listed in Table 3-5 ovarian dose is often used to estimate conceptus dose. (For ovarian doses see Kereiakes and Rosenstein, 1980.) Hŭsák and Wiedermann (1980) have shown that there can be substantial error (40% to 90% too low) in using these estimates for radionuclides excreted through the bladder. This is because of the proximity of the bladder to the uterus. These estimates also do not account for possible placental transfer of the radionuclide.

Once the dose to the conceptus has been approximated by qualified personnel, we proceed to ask the following question.

> ## What is the conception age?

Note: All ages are in *weeks postconception.*
Three methods are employed to determine the gestation age. These are

1. Menstrual history
2. Physical examination
3. Ultrasound

MENSTRUAL HISTORY

Prior to the sixth conception week, gestation age is best determined by an accurate menstrual history. This should include (1) the age of menarche, (2) the regularity and number of days between each period, (3) the usual duration of each menstruation, (4) the amount of flow of the last period, and (5) a history of the recent use of oral contraceptives.

Ovulation occurs approximately 14 days prior to the beginning of each menstrual period. On the basis of an accurate menstrual history, a woman with a 35-day menstrual cycle whose last menstrual period (LMP) began January 1 would be 4 weeks postconception as of February 19. On the other hand, a woman with a 21-day cycle whose LMP began January 1 would be 6 weeks postconception on February 19.

The normal duration of each menstrual cycle and the usual amount of flow are important because many women will have a menstrual-like episode at the time of placental implantation (Hartmann's placental sign). This is often confused for a light period by pregnant women and occurs in around 15% of all pregnancies.

The regularity of the menstrual cycle is important because many women who have an anovulatory cycle may appear to be further along in pregnancy than is actually the case. This is due to the fact that menstruation often does not follow anovulatory cycles.

An oral contraceptive history should be elicited, since long-standing use may lead to anovulatory cycles for 1 or 2 months after the oral contraceptives are stopped.

PHYSICAL EXAMINATION

Figure 6-1 shows the progressive enlargement of the uterus in the first trimester as well as the fundal height increase throughout the entire duration of the pregnancy. There is very little difference between a nongravid uterus and a gravid one before the fourth week postconception. However, between the sixth and eighth weeks postconception there is a palpable increase in uterine size. At 10 weeks postconception the fundus extends above the symphysis pubis. After the 16th week, the centimeter height of the fundus above the symphysis generally corresponds to the conception age in weeks (McDonald's rule).

FIG. 6-1.   The relationship between uterine size and gestational age. (Adapted from Iffy L: Modern Medicine Ob-Gyn Guide, 3rd ed. New York, HBJ Health Care Publications, 1981)

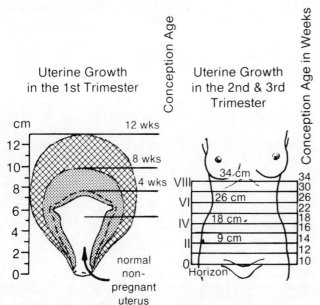

ULTRASOUND

Ultrasound demonstrates intrauterine pregnancy as early as 3 to 4 weeks postconception by identifying the gestational sac within the uterus with a chorionic reaction (gestational ring) around it. A fetal pole may be identified, but no fetal cardiac activity is detected in many cases. By 5 weeks, the embryo is definitely identified, and the fetal cardiac activity is clearly visible. After the sixth week postconception, ultrasound is the most accurate means for determining gestation age. From the sixth to the tenth week, the crown–rump length (CRL) most accurately determines the age. The predicted conception date determined by the CRL differs from that determined by an accurate menstrual history by only 2 or 3 days.

After the 10th week postconception, the fetus can extend and flex its trunk. This compromises the ability of ultrasound to image the entire CRL and renders such measurements unreliable. Beginning at the 11th conception week, the biparietal diameter and the femur length should be used. The biparietal diameter is probably the most accurate measurement of fetal age through the 22nd week postconception.

Table 6-1 correlates ultrasound measurements with conception ages. The table is structured around three critical stages for radiation-induced effects:

Table 6-1. *Conception Age from 6 to 17 Weeks Derived by Ultrasound Parameters*[*]

Conception Age (weeks postconception)	Crown Rump Length[a] (mm)	Femur Length[b] (mm)	Biparietal Diameter[c] (mm)
6	17[d]		
7	24[d]		
8	33[d]		
9	43[d]		
10	54[d]	8[f]	19[e]
11		11[f]	23[e]
12		14[f]	27[e]
13		18[f]	30[e]
14		21[f]	33[e]
15		24[f]	37[e]
16		27[f]	40[f]
17		30[f]	43[f]

[*]Accurate menstrual history required prior to the sixth conception week
[a]Metreweli (1978)
[b]Hadlock and co-workers (1982a)
[c]Hadlock and co-workers (1982b)
[d]95% confidence interval is ±0.5 weeks (rounded to nearest 0.5 weeks)
[e]95% confidence interval is ±1.0 weeks (rounded to nearest 0.5 weeks)
[f]95% confidence interval is ±1.5 weeks (rounded to nearest 0.5 weeks)

from 2 to 7 weeks; between 8 and 15 weeks; and greater than 15 weeks (see Table 4-2). Because of the normal variation in the correlation of these values with conception age, there is a confidence interval that introduces some uncertainty into the evaluation of conceptus age. A more accurate determination can be made if the measurements are repeated in 1 week to 10 days, and they correlate with the previous data.

This information is necessary to ascertain the types of risks to the conceptus. Once the information is acquired, we ask the following question.

What are the radiation risks?

Reasonably suspected risks include possible childhood cancer, small head size, malformation, mental retardation, and resorption of the conceptus. Although diagnostic levels of radiation may be capable of inducing such effects in humans, the likelihood is usually small. Table 4-2 summarizes the possible incidence of these effects as a function of dose and gestation age. Other risks may be associated with radionuclide studies (see Chap. 4, Other forms of malformations).

The job is not yet complete. We proceed to the next question.

What are the risks of not performing the examination?

While the risk of exposing the conceptus to radiation is a primary consideration, the risk of postponing or not performing the radiologic examination must also be considered. The health of the mother is of primary importance and, where serious illness is suspected, this takes priority in determining the need for study. The most important consideration is the effect of defining or not identifying the pathologic process.

A clinical illustration of this would be a woman admitted with severe hyperemesis gravidarum at 6 weeks menstrual age. She develops abdominal pain, low-grade fever, and shoulder pain. Supine and upright films of the abdomen, with shielding of the pelvis, may be required to rule out intestinal obstruction and possible ruptured viscus.

In addition, there is a more subtle risk in not performing an examination when there is a substantial likelihood that the study will be needed later in pregnancy. For example, postponing a radiographic examination during the second week postconception may eliminate the possibility of resorption. However, if the patient's condition deteriorates and the examination is required during the 10th postconception week, the risk of mental retardation becomes a consideration. Planning a radiologic study in light of the conceptual growth pattern can, therefore, be useful in some settings. This issue is discussed in greater detail in Chapter 7.

References

Hadlock FP, Harrist RB, Deter RL et al: Fetal femur length as a predictor of menstrual age: Sonographically measured. Am J Roent 138:875, 1982a

Hadlock FP, Deter RL, Harrist RB et al: Fetal biparietal diameter: A critical re-evaluation of the relation to a menstrual age by means of real time ultrasound. J Ultrasound Med 1:97, 1982b

Hůsák V, Wiedermann M: Radiation absorbed dose estimates to the embryo from some nuclear medicine procedures. Eur J Nucl Med 5:205, 1980

Iffy L: Modern Medicine Ob-Gyn Guide, 3rd ed. New York, HBJ Health Care Publications, 1981

Kereiakes JG, Rosenstein M: Handbook of Radiation Doses in Nuclear Medicine and Diagnostic X Ray. Boca Raton, Florida, CRC Press, 1980

Metreweli C: Practical Clinical Ultrasound. Chicago, William Heinemann, 1978

Chapter 7
Stage III
To Proceed or
Not to Proceed

> ## Should the study be delayed or an
> ## alternative study be considered?

In order to address this question, it is useful to separate patients into two categories: (1) those who may be pregnant, and (2) those who are known to be pregnant.

POSSIBLY PREGNANT PATIENTS

For those patients in the first category, some physicians choose to adhere to the "10-day rule" for examinations involving exposure to the abdomen or pelvis. As Carmichael and Warrick (1978) point out, this "does not truly represent a hard and fast rule and would be better referred to as the '10-day principle.' " In 1972, Great Britain incorporated this into its code of practice (Radioactive Substances Advisory Committee, 1972). The International Commission on Radiation Protection (ICRP, 1970) describes this principle as follows:

> . . . the 10-day interval following the onset of menstruation is the time when it is most improbable that such women (those of reproductive capacity) could be pregnant. Therefore, it is recommended that all radiologic examinations of the lower abdomen and pelvis of women of reproduction capacity that are not of importance in connection with immediate illness of

the patient be limited to this period when pregnancy is improbable. *The examinations that will be appropriate to delay until the onset of the next menstruation are the few that could without detriment be postponed until the conclusion of a pregnancy, or at least until its latter half.*

The goal of this principle is to prevent unnecessary radiation exposure to the conceptuses of women not known to be pregnant. This rule is particularly important if the patient's complaint may be due to an unconfirmed pregnancy. Thus, both the patient and her conceptus are saved unnecessary radiation.

Brown and co-workers (1976a) point out that a too rigorous implementation of this principle may be counterproductive. First, it will delay needed studies for many nonpregnant women, and this may be detrimental to their health care. Second, the authors state that "delaying an examination during this time period will only confront the physician with a decision once the pregnancy is established to conduct the exam during major organogenesis, to delay until fetal stages, until after birth, or to eliminate the exam entirely." If the study were not delayed, the risks are a slight increase in the naturally high incidence of spontaneous abortion and perhaps a small increase in the risk of childhood cancer. Furthermore, there exists some evidence correlating preconception irradiation to an increased incidence of leukemia (Graham et al, 1966). Based on this possibility and the potential genetic risks associated with ionizing radiation, Brown and co-workers suggest there is no interval during which a radiologic study on a woman is completely free of risk to her future offspring. The position of Brown (1976b) and the American College of Radiology regarding the 10-day principle is

Abdominal radiologic examinations that have been requested after *full* consideration of the clinical status of the patient, including the possibility of pregnancy, need not be postponed or selectively scheduled, except in those infrequent instances where the examination may not be related to the patient's current illness.

The wording is similar to that in the recommendation of the ICRP (1970) cited earlier.

Carmichael and Warrick (1978) point out that the data of Graham and associates (1966) is tenuous. A subsequent report by Kneale and Stewart (1980) finds no evidence for an increased risk of leukemia from preconception x rays. Carmichael and Warrick agree that "application of the 10-day principle does not necessarily involve the postponement of all nonurgent abdominal and pelvic radiologic examinations of women presenting in the second half of the menstrual cycle." They do suggest that there are studies needed for a current problem that can be delayed until term.

Both positions are consistent with the ICRP's recommendation. The only disagreement is in distinguishing those examinations that are promptly needed from those that can be delayed. Both agree that the possibility of pregnancy should be taken into account before a request for an abdominal or pelvic examination is made.

Ellis and co-workers (1977), Langmead (1977), Sear (1978), and Taylor (1979) discuss the application of the "10-day rule" for radionuclide applications. Some believe it should apply whenever gonadal (conceptus) doses exceed 50 mrem, others suggest the lower limit be 500 mrem. The duration and distribution of the radioactivity complicates the application of the rule. If a study is performed within 10 days of a patient's last menstruation, it has been suggested that she delay conception for a period sufficient to reduce the radioactivity of her body to about 5% of the administered value or for 2 months, whichever is longer.

The National Council on Radiation Protection and Measurements (NCRP, 1977) recommends that "if, in the best judgment of the attending physician, a diagnostic examination or nuclear medicine procedure *at that time* is deemed advisable to the medical well-being of the patient, it should be carried out without delay, with special efforts being made, however, to minimize the dose received by the lower abdomen (uterus)."

Regarding nuclear medicine procedures, the NCRP (1982) states, "In view of the findings . . . relating to radiation protection of the fetus and the fact that radiation doses of the order of a few rads may be associated with an increased incidence of leukemia and childhood malignancies, it is important to keep the fetal doses below these levels and to carry out only investigations that are imperative during pregnancy."

The physician contemplating the delay of a study should consider the consequences in view of the possibility that the diagnostic examination might become necessary later in the pregnancy. During the first 2 weeks postconception the risks are possible carcinogenesis and resorption. If the study is delayed, but becomes necessary prior to the eighth week postconception, the risks include congenital malformation and small head size, as well as carcinogenesis. If the study is delayed beyond the 8th week but becomes necessary before the 15th, the risks include small head size, mental retardation, and neoplasm. After the 15th week of conception, the only risk for externally delivered diagnostic radiation is carcinogenesis, which is much reduced from the risk during the first trimester. Although the radiation risks during this period may be at their smallest, the amount of x-radiation required to obtain a radiographic study of the abdomen will increase because of the enlarging patient. In addition, the diagnostic criteria are sometimes compromised by the enlarging conceptus.

As the conceptus develops, placental transfer of radionuclides in nuclear medicine studies becomes an important factor. After the eighth conception week, there are known risks to the fetal thyroid from radioiodine studies.

When the decision is made that a diagnostic evaluation should not be delayed, an alternative but less satisfactory diagnostic study that exposes the potential conceptus to relatively little or no ionizing radiation may be chosen. A less-than-optimal study sometimes proves adequately diagnostic. For example, the preferred diagnostic study for urinary calculi is the intravenous pyelogram (IVP). It provides better definition of calculi and the surrounding anatomy than does ultrasound. However, in some cases ultrasound might provide the necessary diagnostic information. It is important that any alternative procedure deliver substantially less or no ionizing radiation to the conceptus. This ensures that the risks would not be significantly increased if the primary study is still required.

PATIENT KNOWN TO BE PREGNANT

In this case, the consideration is whether to delay the study because of radiation risks associated with the known gestation age. This may be especially important if the patient is known to be between the 8th and 15th weeks postconception, since this is the period of greatest risk for mental retardation. For the patient at an early stage of pregnancy, the consequences of delaying the examination should be considered as discussed in the previous paragraphs. Alternatively, the physician may want to consider other diagnostic studies that use little or no ionizing radiation as discussed in the previous paragraph.

Counsel patient on the risks and benefits

Counseling of the patient and other appropriate persons regarding the risks of and the need for the diagnostic procedure is essential (Shepard, 1983a; Mossman and Hill, 1982). It may be desirable for the husband or other appropriately involved persons to be present during the counseling session. The presence of a female nurse or other medical professional may provide emotional support to the patient and medicolegal substantiation of the physician's statements on the risks and benefits of the procedure. The emotional status, age, and education of the involved parties must be taken into consideration. If the patient is a juvenile, it is appropriate to discuss the matter with her guardians. In some cases, it may be appropriate to discuss the circumstance with relatives so that they can provide the patient with emotional support in the decision-making process.

There are several rules of what not to do in a counseling session. Shepard (1983a) advises

The patient should not be told

1. What cannot be understood
2. What cannot be remembered
3. What cannot be believed.

A statement that may not be understood by the patient is, "The exposed conceptus is 16 times more sensitive to the radiocarcinogenic effects of x rays than adults." Another is, "The baby runs a risk of developing cancer at a rate of two to three times greater per rad than the risk for children not exposed to radiation." These statements provide no perspective and are meaningless without additional information. A more useful statement might be, "Radiation-induced childhood cancer has been associated with children who received diagnostic x rays while in the womb. However, the incidence of such events is rare, and the likelihood that the child will not develop cancer is nearly the same as that for pregnant women who are not exposed to x rays." If the patient is capable of interpreting numbers, some percent likelihoods that the child will not develop cancer may be appropriate (see Table 4-1).

If the explanation is lengthy, the patient may not be able to remember the information. It may be appropriate to write down some of the salient points. These might include the patient's condition, the reason for the study, and the suspected risks, along with the likelihood that such untoward events might occur. In addition, appropriate references can be made available to the patient. These might help in the event that the patient finds the oral counseling difficult to understand.

It is best to impartially and calmly communicate the advantages and risks to the appropriate parties. Time must be allowed for questions and for concerns to be expressed. Shepard advises that the bodily movements and facial expressions of the counseled parties can be used as indicators regarding comprehension of the information. The physician can alter his counseling on the basis of these factors. Telephone conversations are deficient in this regard and may be appropriate only if the risk from the examination is considered very minimal.

To put risks into perspective, the physician should be aware of the normal risks of pregnancy and the multiple teratogenic factors in modern living. Approximately 3% of all children are born with congenital defects that require medical attention (Shepard, 1983a). As many as 6% of all humans have detectable congenital defects. Some defects may result from maternal conditions or from man-made substances. Table 7-1 lists some agents or conditions and associated defects. For a thorough review of teratogens, see Shepard (1983b), Brown and Freehafer (1975), Schardein (1976), and Heinonen and associates (1977).

The counseling session should also include nonradiation risks of the di-

Table 7-1. Agents or Conditions with Associated Risks During Pregnancy

Agent or Condition	Associated Defect(s)
Social	
Alcohol	IUGR,* CNS atrophy
Smoking	IUGR
Illicit drugs	IUGR (malnutrition)
Viral infection	
Rubella	IUGR, deafness, cataracts, heart anomalies
CMV (cytomegalovirus)	IUGR, microcephaly, chorioretinitis, thrombocytopenia
Herpes	IUGR, meningitis, chorioretinitis, thrombocytopenia
Other infection	
Toxoplasmosis	IUGR, brain cyst, retinitis
Syphilis	IUGR, bone deformity, saddle nose
Endocrine disorders	
Diabetes	Hydrocephaly, anencephaly, caudal regression syndrome, stillbirth
Hyper-/Hypothyroidism	Goiter, stillbirth
Phenylketonuria	IUGR, prematurity
Prescribed drugs	
Androgenic hormones (testosterone)	Virilization
Anticonvulsants	Cleft lip/palate, IUGR, fetal hydantoin syndrome
Coumarin	Micrognathia, epiphyseal stippling
Diethylstilbestrol	Vaginal adenosis, uterine deformity
Aminopterin	Immune deficiency
Aspirin	Thrombocytopenia
Tetracycline	Bone deformity
Lithium carbonate	Malformation of heart and great vessels
Accutane (isoprotenoic acid)	Hydrocephaly, microcephaly
Other maternal conditions	
Malnutrition	IUGR
Rh-isoimmunization	Mental retardation, anemia
Advanced maternal age	Trisomy
Genetic	Tay-Sachs disease, trisomies
Spontaneous abortion (35%–62% of all pregnancies)	None

*Intrauterine growth retardation

agnostic procedure. An example is the use of iodinated contrast agents that may cause a reaction. These are usually reviewed by the radiologist. In particular, if an extensive procedure is planned, it is appropriate to have the radiologist counsel the patient.

> **Patient agrees to proceed with study?**

It is the patient's prerogative to decline the examination. The physician should inform the patient of the risks of not performing the procedure.

If the patient agrees to proceed with the diagnostic study, the cardinal link in keeping the risk to her conceptus at a minimum is for the referring physician to talk to the radiologist.

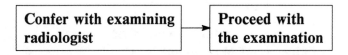

> **Confer with examining radiologist** → **Proceed with the examination**

The radiologist should be informed that the patient is pregnant and why the study is being requested. This can result in several beneficial actions:

- An alternative study involving less radiation may be recommended (see Case Report No. 1, Chap. 11).
- It may be possible to limit the examination to a less than standard procedure while acquiring the necessary information.
- The radiologist might shield the uterus or otherwise avoid inadvertent exposure to the uterine area.
- The most x-ray–efficient radiographic equipment available can be selected for the study.
- The radiologist might decide to remove the grid during fluoroscopy (Gray and Swee, 1982).
- For radionuclide imaging it may be practical to decrease the usual amount of radioactivity for the study and compensate by increasing imaging time.

Perreault and co-workers (1982) discuss the use of a limited radiologic examination for the pregnant patient with symptoms of urinary calculi. Spontaneous elimination of the calculi may obviate the need for x-ray examination. In some cases, however, a pyelographic examination may be desirable. The radiologist might consider limiting the study to two exposures, one prior to injection of contrast material and one approximately 30 minutes later.

When proceeding with an examination on a patient known to be pregnant, a conscientious effort should be made to keep a record of the amount of fluoroscopic exposure time; the number of radiographs, including spot films; the techniques used during fluoroscopy and radiography; and any special circumstances, such as the use of magnification. These factors greatly facilitate the work of the physicist in evaluating conceptus dose.

The physician can consider taking certain actions that help keep the conceptus dose at a minimum. For normal-sized patients with anteverted uteri, anteroposterior (AP) studies deliver about four times more dose than postoroanterior (PA) studies. PA fluoroscopy is the preferred technique for such patients. Only contemporary low-dose image intensified fluoroscopy should be used. The radiologist might choose to do the fluoroscopy without a grid. This would reduce patient dose by a factor of 2 to 8 (Gray and Swee, 1982). For the filming of the study, fast-response film–screen systems should be employed. Such considerations will substantially help to minimize conceptus dose for pregnant patients.

> ### Refer to postexamination flowchart
> ### if patient is pregnant

After the study, the patient may be anxious regarding the amount of radiation received. Sometimes, the patient is not informed of the results of the radiation exposure calculation. It is our belief that sharing this information with the concerned patient is desirable. Referring physicians should consult the postexamination flowchart for the counseling of patients after the examination.

References

Brown A, Freehafer J: Prenatal risks—A pediatrician's point of view. In Aladjem S (ed): Risks in the Practice of Modern Obstetrics, 2nd ed, p 340–358. St. Louis, CV Mosby, 1975

Brown RF, Shaver JW, Lamel DA: A Concept and Proposal Concerning the Radiation Exposure of Women, RHSEP publication No. 874. San Francisco, University of California, 1976a

Brown RF: Prepared Remarks for the October 20, 1976 American College of Radiology Press Conference, Chicago, American College of Radiology, 1976b

Carmichael JHE, Warrick CK: The ten day rule—Principles and practice. Br J Radiol 51:843, 1978

Ellis RE, Nordin BEC, Tothill P et al: The application of the ten day rule in radiopharmaceutical investigations. A report of a working party of the MRC Isotope Advisory Panel. Br J Radiol 50:200, 1977

Graham S, Levin ML, Lilienfield AM et al: Preconception, intrauterine, and postnatal irradiation as related to leukemia. In Haenszel W (ed): Epidemiological Approaches to the Study of Cancer and Other Chronic Diseases. National Cancer Institute Monograph No. 19, pp 347–371. Bethesda, MD, US Department of Health, Education, and Welfare, 1966

Gray JE, Swee RG: The elimination of grids during intensified fluoroscopy and photofluoro spot imaging. Radiology 144:426, 1982

Heinonen OP, Slone B, Shapiro S: Birth Defects and Drugs in Pregnancy. Littleton, Massachusetts, Publishing Sciences Group, 1977

ICRP (International Commission on Radiation Protection): Protection of the Patient in X-ray Diagnosis, publication No. 16. Oxford, Pergamon Press, 1970

Kneale GW, Stewart AM: Preconception x-ray and childhood cancers. Br J Cancer 41:222, 1980

Langmead WA: The application of the "ten-day rule" in radiopharmaceutical investigations. Br J Radiol 50:840, 1977

Mossman KL, Hill LT: Radiation risks in pregnancy. Obstet Gynecol 60:237, 1982

NCRP (National Council on Radiation Protection and Measurements): Medical Radiation Exposure of Pregnant and Potentially Pregnant Women, NCRP report No. 54. Washington, DC, National Council on Radiation Protection and Measurements, 1977

NCRP (National Council on Radiation Protection and Measurements): Nuclear Medicine— Factors Influencing the Choice and Use of Radionuclides in Diagnosis and Therapy, NCRP report No. 70. Washington, DC, National Council on Radiation Protection and Measurements, 1982

Perreault JP, Paquin JM, Foucher R et al: Urinary calculi in pregnancy. Can J Surg 25:453, 1982

Radioactive Substances Advisory Committee: Code of Practice for the Protection of Persons Against Ionizing Radiation Arising from Medical and Dental Use. London, Her Majesty's Stationary Office, 1972

Schardein JL: Drugs as Teratogens. Cleveland, CRC Press, 1976

Sear R: Applicability of the "ten-day rule" to radiopharmaceutical investigations. Br J Radiol 51:58, 1978

Shepard TH: Counseling pregnant women exposed to potentially harmful agents during pregnancy. Clin Obstet Gynecol 26:478, 1983a

Shepard TH: Catalog of Teratogenic Agents, 4th ed. Baltimore, Johns Hopkins Press, 1983b

Taylor DM: Radionuclide investigations in pregnancy—Protection of the embryo and fetus. Br J Radiol 52:605, 1979

Part III
The Clinical Evaluation of Pregnant Patients Previously Exposed to Diagnostic Radiations

PostExamination Flowchart

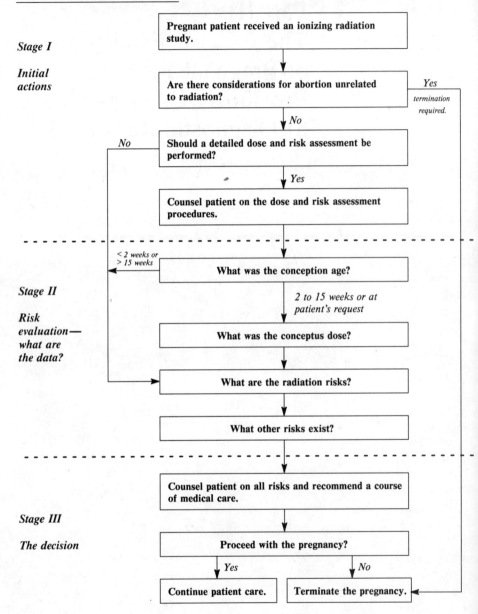

Stage I

*Initial
actions*

Pregnant patient received an ionizing radiation study.

Are there considerations for abortion unrelated to radiation?

Yes

*termination
required.*

No

No

Should a detailed dose and risk assessment be performed?

Yes

Counsel patient on the dose and risk assessment procedures.

*< 2 weeks or
> 15 weeks*

What was the conception age?

Stage II

*Risk
evaluation—
what are
the data?*

*2 to 15 weeks or at
patient's request*

What was the conceptus dose?

What are the radiation risks?

What other risks exist?

Counsel patient on all risks and recommend a course of medical care.

Stage III

The decision

Proceed with the pregnancy?

Yes

No

Continue patient care.

Terminate the pregnancy.

110

Chapter 8
Stage I,
Initial Actions

Pregnant patient received an ionizing radiation study

There can be many reasons why a pregnant patient received an ionizing radiation study. It could have been a planned exposure as discussed in the preexamination flowchart. The exposure might have resulted from an emergency when a thorough evaluation for pregnancy was impractical. Sometimes the pregnancy was unsuspected at the time of the study. Whatever the reason, when presented with a pregnant patient who has received an ionizing radiation study, following is the first question to address.

Are there considerations for abortion unrelated to radiation?

Compromising health circumstances, emotional problems, and attitudes toward the pregnancy that are unrelated to radiation should be brought to the surface and settled. Radiation should not be used as a spurious justification to terminate a pregnancy. If, on the other hand, the parents desire to

111

continue with the pregnancy, the risks from the diagnostic radiation should be assessed as one of the possible compromising health factors. At this point the physician must decide the next question.

> # Should a detailed dose and risk assessment be done?

The decision whether or not to proceed with a detailed dose and risk assessment depends on many factors. These include

1. The conception age at the time of irradiation, if known
2. The conceptus dose, if known, which will depend on
   a) the number and types of studies performed
   b) the type of equipment used
   c) the confidence of the physicians regarding the calibration of the x-ray equipment
   d) the size of the patient
   e) the experience of the physicians in performing dose estimates
3. The emotional state of the patient and whether or not she requests such an evaluation

If the conceptus is known to not have been more than 2 weeks beyond conception or was more than 15 weeks beyond conception, there is little to be gained from an in-depth review of the dose and risks. For the very young conceptus, there are two possible consequences. The first is radiation-induced abortion, in which case the dose received would be irrelevant to future medical care. Current evidence indicates that radiation-induced abnormalities are extremely unlikely, and perhaps zero, for diagnostic irradiation during this time. Another possibility is radiation-induced childhood cancer, but the likelihood that the child would *not* develop cancer is extremely high (see Table 4-1).

For a fetus beyond the 15th week postconception, there appears to be a threshold of 50 rad, below which there is negligible threat of radiation-induced mental retardation. It would be highly unusual for a fetus to receive this amount of radiation from diagnostic studies. We are unaware of any reported incidents of such doses from diagnostic examinations. Unless there are extraordinary circumstances that could lead to such high doses, an in-depth review of dose and risks is not likely to have any consequential influence on the future medical care of the patient, and it is therefore unnecessary.

If the patient is between the 2nd and 15th week postconception, some preliminary rough estimates of conceptus dose should be made to determine whether an in-depth review is necessary. The counseling physician should not rely on the recall of the patient to determine the types of examinations performed. The patient should be queried about all the clinics, hospitals, and physicians' offices she visited. Their records should be checked to see who requested what studies and who performed them. The actual number of completed studies should be verified.

If the experience of the counseling physician and the radiologist(s) in dose evaluation is sufficient to ensure that doses from the radiologic examinations could not have exceeded 1 rad to the conceptus, then there is little to be gained from an in-depth review, regardless of gestation age. No malformation risk has been implicated for human exposures to less than 1 rad, and the cancer risk associated with this level of conceptus dose is extremely small compared to other normal risks of pregnancy.

If the studies included only routine head, extremity, or thoracic examinations, the dose is unlikely to have exceeded 1 rad as long as the studies were properly done (*i.e.,* good radiographic technique was employed). The uterine dose levels from such studies are normally less than 10 mrad. Only extraordinary and virtually unrealistic circumstances in performing these studies could result in radiation levels to a conceptus in excess of 1 rad (*e.g.,* multiple studies on a very large patient using excessively large radiation fields).

A single routine computed tomography (CT) study involving a series of 1-cm slices through the head, thorax, or extremities is also unlikely to result in a conceptus dose exceeding 1 rad.

If the patient received a single upright KUB (kidney–ureter–bladder) or pelvic radiograph, and this was the only abdominal study done, it is unnecessary to do an in-depth dose evaluation unless the calibration of the machine is suspect or other potentially high-dose factors exist, such as obesity and a severely anteverted uterus.

It is not always necessary to perform an in-depth review for CT or fluoroscopic studies in which the uterus was not in the direct x-ray field. Doses from well-designed studies (*e.g.,* a carefully performed upper GI series excluding the pelvis) would normally not exceed 1 rad to the uterus. If, during fluoroscopy, the uterus was only momentarily exposed during the passage of a catheter from the femoral artery to the upper abdomen or thorax, then an in-depth dose evaluation is unnecessary. If there is any reason to suspect higher dose levels (*e.g.,* the study was long because of pathologic findings; the patient was very large; the x-ray equipment was not recently calibrated; the examination included fluoroscopic or radiographic investigation of the lower abdomen), then an in-depth review of dose and risks should be considered. If the counseling physician or radiologist does not have the experience in dose evaluation to make this judgment, a radiological physicist should be consulted.

For nuclear medicine studies, Table 3-5 should be used to roughly estimate dose to the conceptus, keeping in mind the caveats regarding dose evaluations for radionuclide studies (see Chap. 3). This table provides conceptus dose in rad per millicurie activity given the patient. The administered radioactivity should be verified with the department that performed the study before calculating conceptus dose. A table of recommended administered activities should not be used. If the patient was in an early stage of pregnancy and had no difficulty urinating, these dose estimates are the most accurate by today's standards. If there is any uncertainty in performing these calculations, or if the agent does not appear in Table 3-5, or if other complications in dose evaluation arise, consultation with a medical physicist is appropriate.

When the counseling physician decides an in-depth evaluation is not warranted, the patient should be advised of the reasons behind the decision. Other circumstances that may compromise the conceptus should be reviewed along with the normal risks of pregnancy (see last part of "Counsel Patient on Risks and Benefits," Chap. 7). A detailed risk assessment should be considered if the patient requests it, or if conception age at time of exposure was 2 to 15 weeks and the estimated conceptus dose exceeded 1 rad. If the gestation age is unknown and the conceptus dose exceeded 1 rad or is also unknown, a more detailed investigation is advised.

When either the counseling physician recommends a review or the patient requests one, following is the next step.

Counsel patient on the dose and risk assessment procedures

Patients who have received diagnostic studies while pregnant are often alarmed because of emotional perceptions surrounding radiation. The physician should advise the patient at this point of the steps that will be taken for risk assessment and give some preliminary information regarding the risks of diagnostic radiations for pregnant women. The following points should be considered:

1. It is unlikely that radiation from diagnostic radiologic examinations will result in any deleterious effects on the child, but the possibility of a radiation-induced effect cannot be entirely ruled out.
2. The patient should be counseled that this risk assessment is being done, not because there is reason to believe there is grave risk in her circumstance, but simply because these are precautions taken whenever a pregnant woman receives certain diagnostic studies.

3. Each case must be assessed according to the gestational age when exposed and the radiation levels received by the conceptus from each exposure.

4. It is often necessary to obtain the consultation of a physicist to calculate the radiation level received by the baby, and there may be a consultation fee for this.

5. The dose evaluation may take up to a week to complete.

6. When all the information is acquired, the radiation risk will be assessed and will be reviewed along with other possible risks of pregnancy so that the physician, the patient, and other involved persons understand the circumstances and can make reasonable decisions regarding the management of the pregnancy.

Chapter 9
Stage II,
Risk Evaluation—
What Are the Data?

What was the conception age?

Evaluation of conception age is reviewed in Chapter 6 under the section "What is the conception age?"

Conception age is important in risk evaluation for reasons discussed in Chapter 4. In some cases, it may turn out that the patient was less than 2 weeks postconception or not pregnant at the time of the examination. As discussed in Chapter 8, there is little to be gained from a dose evaluation in that situation, because the only risks are possible radiation-induced abortion and perhaps a risk of childhood cancer. Nothing can be done about the possible abortion, and the cancer risks are insufficient to warrant a termination of the pregnancy.

If the conceptus is beyond the 15th week postconception, the only suspected risk from diagnostic levels of radiation would again be possible childhood cancer. The risk would be even less than that for a first-trimester exposure. An in-depth dose evaluation is unnecessary.

If on the other hand, the conception age is determined to have been within the 2nd through 15th weeks postconception, an in-depth dose evaluation is necessary to assess the possibility of radiation-induced small head size, malformation, or mental retardation.

What was the conceptus dose?

If there is an accurate record of the radiation studies performed and the radiation techniques used, then calculation of radiation dose to the conceptus should be straightforward. Descriptions of the calculative methods are provided in the appendices.

The compilation of the data required for dose estimation may be compromised by the recalls of the personnel regarding duration of fluoroscopy, retakes of films, and other factors. In order to obtain a reasonable estimate of the dose, the following guidelines are proposed:

Don't . . .

- Assume that doses from survey charts give the actual dose to your patient. This is not satisfactory because such doses may be 10 times more or less than the actual dose.

Do . . .

1. Review patient records to establish the number of radiologic examinations performed at all institutions that the patient may have visited.
2. Review the film files and document the field size and the following for each film: uterus within field-of-view; uterus adjacent to field-of-view (<10 cm from edge); uterus more than 10 cm from edge of field-of-view. If uterus is in field-of-view, note if it is shielded by bone, barium, or other material.
3. Review with the technologist the computed tomographic and radiographic techniques used, and inquire about the possibility of discarded radiographs. Review fluoroscopy techniques and exposure time.
4. Review with the radiologist the techniques used in fluoroscopy, the use of grids, the use of 4-, 6-, or 9-inch, or other field size, and the duration of fluoroscopy. Inquire about the relative position of the uterus with respect to the fluroscopy field and the duration of fluoroscopy with the uterus in view.
5. Measure the anteroposterior thickness of the patient's pelvis at uterus level. This information is required to determine dose rates in fluoroscopy, x-ray output for automatic exposure-controlled radiography, and source-to-skin distance.
6. Review the ultrasound studies for data valuable to ascertain the depth of the uterus at the time of radiographic examination. If ultrasound is not available, consideration might be given to acquiring such a study if needed. (Conceptus depth measurements may be compromised if the ultrasonographer depresses the abdomen during the study.)

7. Check the calibration of the radiographic equipment used for abdominal examinations. Measure the half-value layer for the kVp used in the studies. Note the entrance exposure to the patient for the radiographic studies. Measure fluoroscopy entrance-dose rate to the patient using information from numbers 3, 4 and 5 in this list and a water bath to simulate patient-thickness. Measure the source-to-image receptor distance and the source-to-tabletop distance.

8. Calculate the conceptus dose using methods described in Appendix A.

9. Obtain records of all nuclear medicine studies to estimate conceptus dose from administered activity of radiopharmaceuticals. Doses may be estimated from data in Table 3-5 with due consideration for uncertainties discussed in Chapter 3. If data from Table 3-5 are insufficient, dose must be estimated from methods outlined in Appendix B or from ovarian doses (see Chap. 6).

10. Judge the accuracy of the calculations. There are several sources of uncertainty, including depth of conceptus; bladder distension; shielding of uterus by bone or barium; patient contour; uniformity of the diagnostic x-ray field; technologist's recall of radiographic exposure techniques and retakes; proximity of the uterus to the x-ray field during fluoroscopy; estimation of the exposure time during fluoroscopy with conceptus in and outside field-of-view; amount of radioactivity administered during radionuclide procedures; and uncertainties in radionuclide procedures regarding frequency of urination and placental transfer of the radionuclide (see Appendices A and B).

Once the information on conceptus dose is acquired, the physician confronts the next question.

What are the radiation risks?

These are outlined in Table 4-2 as a function of dose and gestation age. The consequences of high doses from radionuclides in organs of the conceptus are reviewed in Chapter 4 (section on "Other Forms of Malformations"). Prior to presenting the information to the patient it is important to ascertain a perspective of the situation and to review other risks that may exist.

What other risks exist?

Exposure of the patient to other teratogenic agents should be assessed. Intrauterine growth retardation is associated with smoking and alcohol consumption. The teratogenic risks of medications that the patient may be receiving should be reviewed. The possibility of teratogenesis from infectious agents such as rubella, syphilis, or herpes should be considered. Possible genetic risks are another important factor. Some of these are reviewed in Chapter 7 (see section "Counsel Patient on Risks and Benefits") and in Table 7-1.

Chapter 10
Stage III,
The Decision

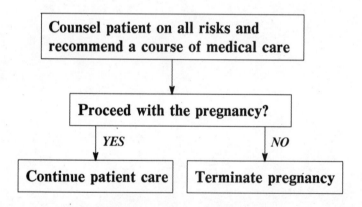

Counseling the patient on risks and benefits of a diagnostic radiologic study and comparing these to the normal risks of pregnancy are discussed in Chapter 7. In this situation, however, the patient has already been exposed to the radiation, and the emotional circumstances may be different.

If the diagnostic study was performed with the foreknowledge of the patient's pregnancy, she may still be apprehensive regarding the actual dose that her conceptus received and the possible risks involved. Postexamination counseling can aid in alleviating anxiety that may linger after the study. If the conceptus did not receive more radiation than anticipated, the patient should be advised of this so she knows that the risks are not greater, and are perhaps less, than previously discussed.

The situation is quite different if the patient received significantly higher levels of radiation than anticipated. If pregnancy was not suspected during examination, still other issues need to be addressed. The patient should be advised of the actual dose received by the conceptus and the radiation risks involved. Other potential or actual risks should be reviewed and placed in their proper perspective. (Suggestions on how to communicate this information to the patient are provided in Chap. 7 in the section "Counsel Patient on Risks and Benefits.") Table 7-1 reviews other teratogenic risks and conditions.

Brent and Gorson (1972) make the following statement regarding therapeutic abortion from diagnostic radiation:

> A decision as to whether to terminate the pregnancy would depend on (1) the hazard of the pregnancy to the expectant mother, (2) the extent and type of radiation hazard to the embryo or fetus, (3) the ethnic and religious background of the family, (4) the laws of the state pertaining to legal abortion, and (5) any other relevant considerations.

We concur with this advice.

It is often the case that patients who receive high doses of radiation from diagnostic studies have other factors compromising the conceptus and the patient. The pregnancy may exacerbate the problem and threaten the mother.

The ethnic and religious background of the parents will significantly affect their response to the clinical advice of the physician. The physician should respect the moral attitudes of the parents and place the medical circumstances into a perspective so that the patient is fully aware of her options and their possible consequences.

Laws regarding abortion in various countries and provinces differ considerably. Radiation exposure to pregnant women for medical reasons should not be used as a spurious legal justification for terminating a pregnancy.

"Other relevant considerations" might include other teratogens to which the patient may have been exposed, or other clinical conditions such as malnutrition, disease, genetic factors, age, and the like.

In 1959, Hammer-Jacobsen established a precedent for the indication of therapeutic abortion from ionizing radiation received for medical purposes. This is often referred to as "The Danish Rule." The suggested guidelines were as follows:

- For doses less than about 1 rad there is no indication for therapeutic abortion.
- If there are additional risk factors involved, therapeutic abortion is advisable for doses between 1 rad and about 10 rad.
- Therapeutic abortion is advised for conceptus doses exceeding 10 rad.

Hammer-Jacobsen encouraged discussion and reevaluation of these guidelines with the disclosure of updated information. In the past 25 years, substantial amounts of new information have been made available (see Chap. 4 and references therein). Based on more recent knowledge, other guidelines have been suggested by various organizations.

The National Council on Radiation Protection (NCRP, 1977) says the following:

> The risk [of abnormality] is considered to be negligible at 5 rad or less when compared to other risks of pregnancy, and the risk of malformations is significantly increased above control levels only at doses above 15 rad. Therefore, exposure of the fetus to radiation arising from diagnostic procedures would very rarely be cause, by itself, for terminating a pregnancy.

The American College of Radiology (Brown, 1976) has taken the following position regarding indication for therapeutic abortion from diagnostic radiation:

> Interruption of pregnancy is *never* justified because of radiation risk to the embryo/fetus from a diagnostic examination. This includes exposure from both abdominal and peripheral examinations.

We recommend the following:

- **If received during or prior to the first 2 weeks postconception**, exposure to diagnostic radiation, by itself, is not an indication for therapeutic abortion.

- **For patients exposed to radiation between the second and eighth conception weeks**, therapeutic abortion based solely on radiation exposure is not advised for doses less than 15 rad, unless there are other compromising factors severely threatening either the mother or conceptus, (*e.g.*, acute viral disease, teratogenic drug use, severe pulmonary hypertension). Doses exceeding 15 rad may be an indication for therapeutic abortion in the presence of less severely compromising factors. However, diagnostic studies rarely result in such dose levels.

- **For conceptuses exposed between the 8th and 15th conception week**, human data suggest that there may be a 0.4% per rad increase in the risk of mental retardation. It is not known whether other factors (*e.g.*, malnutrition) may have contributed to this figure.

  At fetal doses below 5 rad, radiation should be considered only a minor teratogenic factor and does not, by itself, represent a sufficient risk to justify therapeutic abortion.

  For doses between 5 rad and 15 rad, therapeutic abortion is not advisable on the basis of the radiation risk alone. It may be advisable if other compromising circumstances exist.

At doses above 15 rad in this time interval (between 8 and 15 weeks postconception), there is sufficient scientific evidence to support a recommendation for therapeutic abortion based solely on the radiation exposure. However, this does not mean an abortion should necessarily be recommended. At 15 rad, there is about a 6% chance that the child could develop severe mental retardation. Conversely, there is about a 94% chance the child will not suffer such an anomaly. The chance that the child will develop cancer is less than 3%. Conversely, the child has better than a 97% chance of not developing cancer. The chance of having a small head size is approximately 15%, but this does not necessarily affect normal function. Except for possible effects to individual organs from some radionuclide studies, no other risks have been demonstrated. It could be argued from these data that abortion is not justified even at these dose levels. Furthermore, the scientific evidence for radiation-induced mental retardation and cancer at diagnostic levels is not definitive since other data exist that show negative results. The counseling physician and the patient must make the decision based on the available information on risk as well as on other circumstances of the pregnancy.

• **For patients exposed to diagnostic radiation after the 15th conception week**, the pregnancy should be carried to term.

References

Brent RL, Gorson RO: Radiation exposure in pregnancy. Curr Probl Radiol 2:1, 1972

Brown RF: Prepared Remarks for the October 20, 1976, American College of Radiology Press Conference, Chicago, American College of Radiology, 1976

Hammer-Jacobsen E: Therapeutic abortion on account of x-ray examination during pregnancy. Dan Med Bull 6:113, 1959

National Council on Radiation Protection and Measurements (NCRP): Medical Radiation Exposure of Pregnant and Potentially Pregnant Women, NCRP report No. 54. Washington, DC, National Council on Radiation Protection and Measurements, 1977

Chapter 11
Case Reports

Case no. 1

MJ was admitted in her 25th week of pregnancy complaining of gross, painless hematuria. She had an undocumented history of episodic hematuria. She had no prenatal care.

Ultrasound revealed a normal left kidney. The upper pole of the right kidney was dilated by a large, complex mass. The middle and lower collection system was dilated and filled with echogenic material (blood, pus, and the like). The findings were suggestive of papillary necrosis, thought to be tuberculous.

The urologist requested an intravenous pyelogram (IVP) for confirmation. The radiologist advised against the IVP, based on ultrasound findings. Since the intent of any further radiologic investigation was to substantiate the diagnosis of tuberculosis, the radiologist recommended a computed tomography (CT) evaluation of the kidneys. This had the added benefit of minimal direct exposure to the fetus (only the rump was exposed).

CT revealed typical evidence of tuberculosis. The patient was started immediately on therapy. Three months later the AFB culture proved positive.

In this instance, the consultation between the urologist and the radiologist saved the fetus unnecessary radiation exposure by avoiding the IVP. CT examination was the study of choice both for diagnosis and for limiting the radiation dose to the patient. In this case, radiologic evaluation reduced maternal morbidity by establishing the diagnosis, thus permitting prompt therapy. It also reduced the risk of congenital tuberculosis in the fetus.

No dose evaluation for the CT study was performed. This is because the diagnostic dose during the third trimester would not warrant any change in the medical care of the patient.

The patient delivered a full-term, normal child.

Case no. 2

CP was a 23-year-old gravida 3, para 2, in her 31st week of pregnancy, with complaints of severe right flank pain, nausea, and vomiting of 1-week duration. Symptomatic therapy had been ineffective. Complete blood count was 12,300 with 84 seg, and hemaglobin 11.5 grams. Differential diagnosis included kidney infection and kidney stone. Ultrasound examination showed bilateral hydronephrosis, right more than left, with no evidence of lithiasis. Urine cultures were negative. After 6 additional days of symptomatic therapy, the pain, nausea, and vomiting persisted.

The attending physician initially suggested that an IVP be performed. The patient was told by her doctor that the child might develop childhood cancer from the exposure, but the likelihood of such an occurrence was not explained. The patient refused the study on the basis of this limited information.

A radiation physicist was then asked to perform a risk evaluation for this patient. The fetal dose was estimated at less than 1 rad per film for a 36-cm-thick abdomen. The 5-cm depth dose was 2.7 rad per film, the 10-cm depth dose was 1.1 rad per film, and the 15-cm depth dose was 0.5 rad per film. (It is significant to note that if the enlarged abdomen of pregnancy had not been taken into account, the dose estimate would have been a factor 5 to 10 less, because thin patients require much less radiation than thick patients [see Chap. 3].)

The radiologist was then asked to discuss the circumstance with the patient and to advise her of the need for the diagnostic study. Considering the patient's fears regarding the cancer risks, it was deemed advisable to ask a radiologist who had recently given birth to her first child to discuss the risks and benefits with the patient. The patient was advised that the risk of childhood cancer was extremely small and that the likelihood her child would not develop cancer was greater than 99%. She was also advised that the study was necessary in order to determine whether surgical intervention would be required to prevent further complications that could result from her kidney ailment. The patient's anxiety was allayed, and she requested that the study be performed as soon as possible.

A limited excretory pyelogram composed of four abdominal films was performed. The examination showed marked hydronephrosis and dilation of the ureter to lower levels with slightly decreased excretion on the right. The afternoon of the examination the patient passed two bits of material she described as "small, bloody clots." The urine was not strained, and the material was not recovered. Following passage of this material the symptoms promptly resolved and did not recur.

The quantity of radiation received by the fetus was discussed with the patient. The very small risk was again discussed. Routine prenatal care was continued and she delivered a normal 3.3-kg (7 lb 4 oz) baby girl.

The goal of the radiologic examination in this case was to ascertain whether or not surgical intervention was indicated. The IVP both contraindicated surgery and may have helped flush the stones. In retrospect, the number of films acquired during this study could have been reduced to two as discussed in Chapter 7.

POSTEXAMINATION CASES

Case no. 3

LS is a 35-year-old primagravida. She was initially seen complaining of abdominal pain. At this time it was discovered that she was approximately 7 weeks pregnant. In addition, she was overweight and was found to have uncontrolled diabetes. During the course of her workup, it was learned that approximately 5 weeks previously she underwent a chest examination at another clinic, where elevation of the right hemidiaphragm was noted. Fluoroscopic examination of the diaphragm was performed by the radiologist. Following this, she went to a local hospital where two posteroanterior (PA) chest radiographs and one lateral radiograph were made. Thirteen days later, an additional PA radiograph and lateral radiograph were exposed. The next day two supine radiographs of the abdomen and one upright radiograph were made. On admission to another hospital, a PA radiograph and a lateral radiograph of the chest were acquired.

The patient was advised that the dose evaluation of a physicist would be required in order to ascertain the radiation risks. She was also advised that it was rare that such risks by themselves would be of sufficient magnitude to warrant interruption of a pregnancy. However, no definitive statement would be possible until such a dose evaluation was complete.

Ultrasound revealed a severely anteverted uterus (6-cm depth to pregnancy and anteroposterior thickness of 26 cm). It was verified that the transducer was not pressed into the abdomen during the study, and so the measurement was not artifactual. The dose to the conceptus was estimated at 2.6 rad, with an upper limit of 5 rad. Note that even a 2.6-rad estimate is unusually high for these examinations. This was due to the anteverted uterus of this large patient.

The diabetes was stabilized with insulin. The patient was counseled about the various risks (age, obesity, diabetes, radiation). She was reassured that the radiation received by the fetus resulted in a small additional risk that, by itself, did not warrant termination of her pregnancy. Because this was her first pregnancy after 10 years of attempting to become pregnant, she was eager to continue with it. The obstetrician recommended continuation, but advised her of all the risks associated with her conditions.

She delivered a full-term 4.4-kg (9 lb 11 oz) baby boy by cesarean section. The child was classified as normal at birth.

Case no. 4

SS was a 16-year-old patient admitted with symptoms of gallbladder disease. Menstrual history did not suggest pregnancy. The patient received a complete upper and lower GI radiographic evaluation consisting of multiple radiographs of the pelvis and a considerable amount of fluoroscopy. The patient also received a nuclear radiologic study involving 5 mCi of ^{99m}Tc PIPIDA. All diagnostic findings were negative. The pregnancy was discovered after ultrasonic study of the pelvis. Dose to the conceptus was estimated at a maximum of 5 rad. This included a 1.3-rad upper-limit dose from the nuclear radiologic study, based on manufacturers' estimates of ovarian dose. The patient was approximately 4 weeks postconception when these studies were performed.

The patient and her parents were advised that her complaints were diagnosed as resulting from pregnancy. At that time, the patient decided to continue with her pregnancy. The patient and parents were counseled that the risks to the child from the radiation received were small compared to the normal risks of the pregnancy. Afterward the patient reconsidered and, for reasons not associated with the radiation, elected to terminate the pregnancy.

Case no. 5

SR was a 17-year-old, 39-kg (85-lb) patient with a 5-year history of systemic lupus erythematosus. She was admitted with lower abdominal pain. A menstrual history did not suggest pregnancy. A fluoroscopic barium enema examination was performed consisting of approximately 4½ minutes of fluoroscopy time, three 105 mm spot films, and seven 36 cm × 43 cm radiographic films. The patient had an IVP examination consisting of four films. She also had two chest examinations, and a CT examination of the head consisting of 16 slices. The latter was performed to ascertain if her disease had infiltrated the cerebrum, because she showed symptoms of depression and malnutrition, and she refused to eat. Intravenous feeding was initiated. She was subsequently diagnosed as pregnant. The conception age at the time of the radiographic studies was about 8 weeks. The conceptus dose from her radiographic studies was estimated at approximately 3 rad.

The parents were advised that the radiation received from the diagnostic studies, by itself, did not present a significant risk to the conceptus. However, in conjunction with her malnutrition and her refusal to eat, the patient and her parents were advised that there was a cause for concern.

The patient and her parents opted for continuation of the pregnancy. During labor, she was taken to the operating room for primary cesarean section for fetal distress. This resulted in a delivery of a baby girl weighing 2 kg (4.4 lbs) and classified as normal at birth.

Appendices

Appendix A
Conceptus Dose Calculations for X-ray Examinations

A quantitative estimation of conceptus dose from x-ray examinations can be separated into two categories: (1) dose when the conceptus is in the direct field-of-view, and (2) dose when the conceptus is outside the field-of-view and is exposed only to scatter radiation. These two categories may be applied to all forms of radiography, including fluoroscopy, digital radiography, and computed tomography. The following sections review calculative methods for estimating conceptus dose. Digital, fluoroscopic, and conventional radiography are all classified as *wide field-of-view radiography* and are treated separately from computed tomography.

In-Field Dose Calculations for Wide Field-of-View Radiography

Before describing each of the four popular techniques used to estimate dose from direct radiographic exposure of a conceptus, some comments on exposure calibration of radiographic equipment are warranted. Parameters important to calibration include

- kVp—the peak kilovoltage applied across the x-ray tube
- waveform—the time dependence of the applied kilovoltage waveform (single-phase or three-phase)

131

- filtration—the materials located inside the x-ray tube housing that prevent the very low energy x rays from reaching the patient, usually measured as an *aluminum equivalent* (see Chap. 3)
- HVL—the quality or half-value layer of the x-ray beam. This is an indirect measure of filtration. It is the amount of aluminum that, when placed in front of the x-ray beam, reduces its exposure intensity to one half its initial value. HVL must be measured using proper geometry (Gray et al, 1983).
- HVT—half-value thickness, same as HVL
- mAs—mA is the x-ray tube current in milliamperes that is used to produce and control the intensity of the x rays. The s is the duration of the x-ray exposure measured in seconds. The product of mA and s is the mAs and is related to the number of x rays used for an exposure.
- mA · min—mA times exposure duration in minutes
- mR/mAs—the exposure output in milliroentgens per unit mAs. It is usually measured at 40" ($\sim$1 m) from the point of x-ray production.
- R/(mA · min)—the exposure output in roentgens per unit mA · min

Most dose-evaluation techniques require that kVp and either the HVL or the filtration be specified. HVL and the filtration are related. The relationship depends on the waveform and the kVp. Table A-1 tabulates the relationship for single-phase equipment. For three-phase equipment, the data are given in Table A-2. These tables are useful if filtration is unknown but is required for use of a calculative technique. HVL can be measured and converted to the proper filtration using the appropriate table.

Table A-1. *Half-Value Layers as a Function of Filtration and Tube Potential for Single-Phase Diagnostic Units*

Total Filtration mm Al	Peak Potential (kV)									
	30	40	50	60	70	80	90	100	110	120
	Typical half-value layers in millimeters of aluminum									
0.5	0.36	0.47	0.58	0.67	0.76	0.84	0.92	1.00	1.08	1.16
1.0	0.55	0.78	0.95	1.08	1.21	1.33	1.46	1.58	1.70	1.82
1.5	0.78	1.04	1.25	1.42	1.59	1.75	1.90	2.08	2.25	2.42
2.0	0.92	1.22	1.49	1.70	1.90	2.10	2.28	2.48	2.70	2.90
2.5	1.02	1.38	1.69	1.95	2.16	2.37	2.58	2.82	3.06	3.30
3.0		1.49	1.87	2.16	2.40	2.62	2.86	3.12	3.38	3.65
3.5		1.58	2.00	2.34	2.60	2.86	3.12	3.40	3.68	3.95

Derived from Hale (1966) by interpolation and extrapolation. (National Council on Radiation Protection and Measurements: Medical Radiation Exposure of Pregnant and Potentially Pregnant Women, report No. 54, p 17. Washington, DC, National Council on Radiation Protection and Measurements, 1977)

Table A-2. **Half-Value Layers as a Function of Filtration and Tube Potential for Three-Phase Diagnostic Units**[a]

Total Filtration mm Al	Peak Potential (kV)								
	60	**70**	**80**	**90**	**100**	**110**	**120**	**130**	**140**
	Half-value layers in millimeters of aluminum								
2.5[b,c]	2.2	2.4	2.7	3.1	3.3	3.6	4.0		
3.0[c]	2.3	2.6	3.0	3.3	3.6	4.0	4.3	4.6	5.0
3.5[b,c]	2.6	2.9	3.2	3.6	3.9	4.3	4.6		

[a](National Council on Radiation Protection and Measurements: Medical Radiation Exposure of Pregnant and Potentially Pregnant Women, report No. 54, p 17. Washington, DC, National Council on Radiation Protection and Measurements, 1977)
[b]Estimated from NCRP (1968)
[c]Kelley and Trout (1971)

All conceptus dose evaluations require that x-ray output at some point in space be estimated for the radiographic techniques used during the examination. These may be measured directly by a physicist (see Chap. 9), or, in some circumstances, they may be estimated from charts. The latter is practical if manual techniques are used because the mAs for each radiograph will be known. Figures A-1 and A-2 graph the exposure output in mR/mAs at 40 inches (~1 m) as a function of kVp and filtration for single- and three-phase equipment with various degrees of filtration. The exposure output at other distances from the source can be obtained using a simple inverse-square-law correction:

$$M\,(h) = M\,(h') \times \frac{(h')^2}{(h)^2} \qquad (A\text{-}1)$$

where $M\,(h')$ is the exposure output measured at distance h' from the source, *and* $M\,(h)$ is the exposure output at distance h from the source.

The exposure in mR at any distance, h, from the source can be calculated by multiplying the output in mR/mAs by the known mAs and correcting for distance using the inverse-square law. However, it should be remembered that it is always more reliable to measure exposure directly rather than to rely on data from published tables and figures.

For fluoroscopy, the output in roentgen per mA · min is given in Table A-3 as a function of kVp, distance from the source, and filtration. This table may be used cautiously to estimate output from equipment. A more accurate dose estimate can be obtained by measuring dose rates under simulated conditions using the equipment employed in the study.

Several techniques have been developed to estimate dose when the conceptus is directly exposed (Ragozzino et al, 1981; Harrison, 1981; Kelley

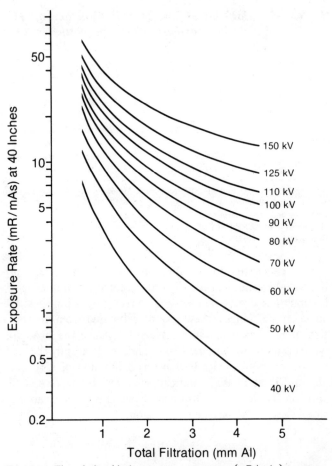

FIG. A-1. The relationship between exposure rates (mR/mAs) versus total filtration and kVp for single-phase full wave rectification. (McCullough EC, Cameron JR: Exposure rates of diagnostic x-ray units. Br J Radiol 43:448, 1978)

and Trout, 1971; Schulz and Gignac, 1976; Sabel et al, 1980; Rosenstein, 1976a, 1976b). Each technique requires that certain data be acquired prior to dose calculation. We describe these techniques here. Added to the dose equations for some techniques are inverse-square correction terms that adjust the calculations for the clinically applicable focal spot-to-patient distances. These terms do not always appear in the original literature and are set off by brackets in this text. Examples using each technique are given at the end of this section.

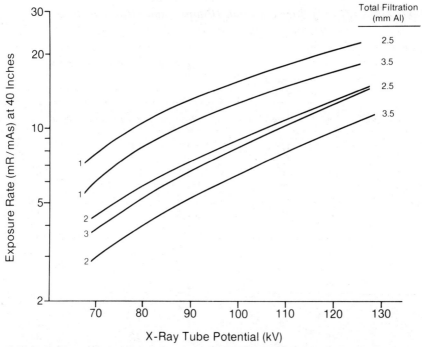

FIG. A-2. The relationship of exposure rate (mR/mAs) versus x-ray tube potential and filtration. Curves 1 (Schulz and Gignac, 1976) were obtained with an x-ray source that showed intensity fluctuations of ± 15% about the mean (3 phase). Curves 2 (NCRP, 1968) were calculated for single-phase full wave rectification. Curve 3 is a graphic representation of single-phase data tabulated by NCRP (1968). (Schulz RJ, Gignac CE: Application of tissue–air ratios for patient doses in diagnostic radiology. Radiology 120:687, 1976)

NORMALIZED DEPTH-DOSE TECHNIQUE
(RAGOZZINO ET AL, 1981)

The conceptus dose in rad per roentgen free-in-air entrance exposure as a function of depth inside the mother is given in Figures A-3 through A-6. The constraints under which the data were acquired include

1. Field size was 36 × 43 cm, with long axis parallel to body.
2. Data in Figures A-3 and A-5 were acquired at 2.5 cm inferior to central axis of x-ray beam.
3. Data in Figures A-4 and A-6 were acquired at 5.1 cm inferior to central axis of x-ray beam.
4. Alderson-Rando phantom was used in all measurements. (Alderson Research Laboratories, Inc., Stanford, CT 06904)

(*Text continues on p 141*)

Table A-3. Effect of Tube Potential, Distance, and Filtration on Air Exposure Rate at Panel of Fluoroscopes

Potential kVp	Source to panel distance cm	inches	1 mm	2 mm	2.5 mm	3 mm	4 mm
			Roentgens per milliampere minute				
70	30	12	5.3	2.7	2.2	1.8	1.3
	38	15	3.5	1.7	1.4	1.2	0.8
	46	18	2.4	1.2	1.0	0.8	0.6
80	30	12	7.0	3.9	3.2	2.6	2.0
	38	15	4.6	2.5	2.1	1.7	1.3
	46	18	3.2	1.8	1.4	1.2	0.9
90	30	12	9.0	5.2	4.3	3.6	2.8
	38	15	5.8	3.3	2.8	2.3	1.8
	46	18	4.0	2.3	1.9	1.6	1.2
100	30	12	11.0	6.6	5.5	4.7	3.7
	38	15	7.0	4.2	3.5	3.0	2.3
	46	18	4.9	2.9	2.5	2.1	1.6
110	30	12	13.1	8.0	6.8	5.9	4.6
	38	15	8.4	5.1	4.4	3.8	3.0
	46	18	5.8	3.5	3.0	2.6	2.0
120	30	12	14.7	9.3	8.0	7.0	5.5
	38	15	9.5	6.0	5.1	4.5	3.6
	46	18	6.5	4.1	3.6	3.1	2.5
130	38	15		6.8	5.9	5.2	4.2
	46	18		4.7	4.1	3.6	2.9
140	38	15		7.6	6.6	5.9	4.8
	46	18		5.3	4.6	4.1	3.3
150	38	15		8.5	7.5	6.7	5.4
	46	18		5.8	5.2	4.6	3.7

(Column header span: "Equivalent total aluminum filtration" covers 1 mm, 2 mm, 2.5 mm, 3 mm, 4 mm)

Typical exposure rates produced by equipment with medium-length cables, derived from Trout and Kelley (1964) and Hale (1966) by interpolation and extrapolation. Filtration includes that of the tabletop and the x-ray tube with its inherent and added filter. As used above, panel means either panel or tabletop. (National Council on Radiation Protection and Measurements: Medical X-ray and Gamma-ray Protection for Energies up to 10Mev, report No. 33, p 42. Washington, DC, National Council on Radiation Protection and Measurements, 1968)

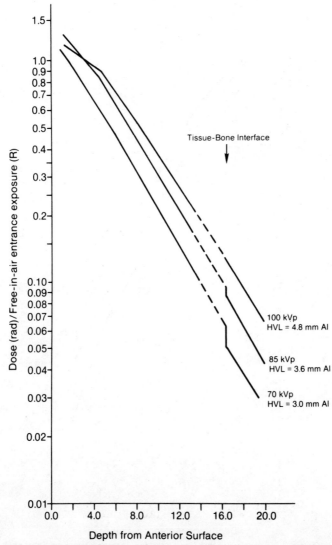

FIG. A-3. Normalized depth-dose data for anteroposterior radiographic field located 2.5 cm inferior to central axis of x-ray beam with a field size of 36 cm × 43 cm. (Redrawn from Ragozzino MW, Gray JE, Burk TM et al: Estimation and minimization of fetal absorbed dose: Data from common radiographic examinations. Am J Roentgenol 137:667, © 1981, American Roentgen Ray Society)

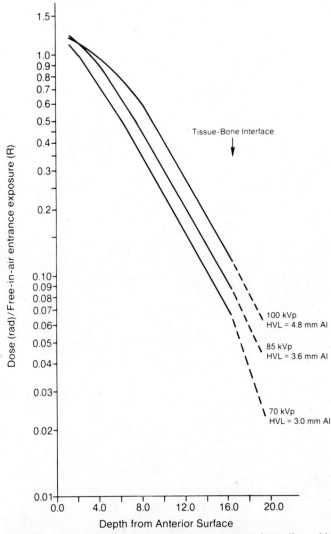

FIG. A-4. Normalized depth-dose data for anteroposterior radiographic field located 5.1 cm inferior to central axis of x-ray beam with a field size of 36 cm × 43 cm. (Redrawn from Ragozzino MW, Gray JE, Burk TM et al: Estimation and minimization of fetal absorbed dose: Data from common radiographic examinations. Am J Roentgenol 137:667, © 1981, American Roentgen Ray Society)

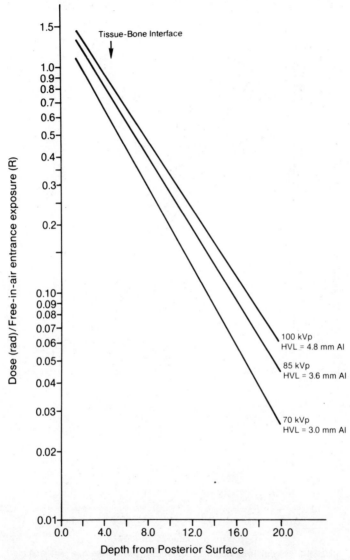

FIG. A-5. Normalized depth-dose data for posteroanterior radiographic field located 2.5 cm inferior to central axis of x-ray beam with a field size of 36 cm × 43 cm. (Redrawn from Ragozzino MW, Gray JE, Burk TM et al: Estimation and minimization of fetal absorbed dose: Data from common radiographic examinations. Am J Roentgenol 137:667, © 1981, American Roentgen Ray Society)

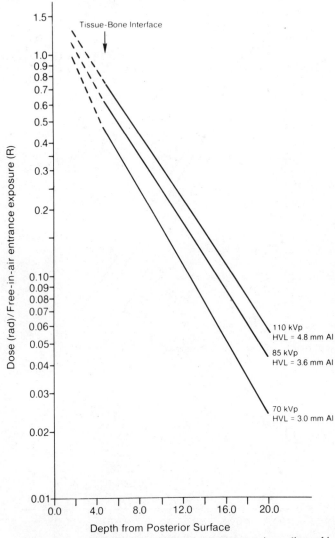

FIG. A-6. Normalized depth–dose data for posteroanterior radiographic field located 5.1 cm inferior to central axis of x-ray beam with a field size of 36 cm × 43 cm. (Redrawn from Ragozzino MW, Gray JE, Burk TM et al: Estimation and minimization of fetal absorbed dose: Data from common radiographic examinations. Am J Roentgenol 137:667, © 1981, American Roentgen Ray Society)

5. Distance from x-ray source to phantom surface was 102 cm.
6. Half-value layer (type 1100 Al) of 70 kVp beam was 3 mm Al.
7. Half-value layer of 85 kVp beam was 3.6 mm Al.
8. Half-value layer of 110 kVp beam was 4.9 mm Al.
9. Waveform was not specified but was similar to three-phase.
10. Added filtration was 5 mm Al.
11. Absolute error of measurements was $\pm 10\%$.

To use this technique, the following data are required for each radiographic exposure:

1. kVp
2. HVL
3. Source exit distance, which is the distance from x-ray source to surface where beam exits the patient
4. Patient AP thickness over position of conceptus
5. Depth of conceptus
6. Free-in-air entrance exposure at skin surface for radiographic conditions used in examination

The absorbed dose to the conceptus is given by

$$D^{(RGB)} = N \cdot X \cdot \left[\frac{(S - L)^2}{(S - L + d)^2} \cdot \left(1 + \frac{d}{102 \text{ cm}}\right)^2 \right] \quad (A\text{-}2)$$

where

- $D^{(RGB)}$ is the conceptus dose in rad (RGB refer to the authors whose data are used here)
- d is the depth (cm) of the conceptus from the entrance surface
- N is the normalized dose for depth d in rad/roentgen
- X is the free-in-air entrance exposure in roentgen
- S is the source exit distance in cm
- L is the AP thickness in cm

Disadvantages of this technique are that it is difficult to extrapolate to half-value layers less than 3 mm, and it does not account for variations in field size.

PERCENTAGE DEPTH-DOSE TECHNIQUE (HARRISON, 1981; KELLEY AND TROUT, 1971)

The relative percentage of dose as a function of depth in the patient for a wide range of field sizes, kVp's, and HVL's is given in Tables A-4 through A-8 and Figures A-7 and A-8. The entrance dose at the surface of the patient is assigned a value of 100%. The constraints for the collection of these data include

(*Text continues on p 147*)

Table A-4. Percentage Depth Doses: 1 mm Al HVT

Depth (cm)	Field Size (cm^2)					
	0	7 × 7	10 × 10	15 × 15	20 × 20	30 × 30
			60 kV$_p$			
0	100	100	100	100	100	100
1	54.0	63.0	68.6	69.3	69.4	69.5
2	34.0	41.0	43.0	43.0	45.0	46.0
3	20.3	28.0	29.5	30.2	31.7	32.1
4	13.0	20.0	21.0	22.0	23.0	24.0
5	8.3	13.8	15.0	16.2	16.7	16.8
6	5.5	9.6	10.8	12.0	12.2	12.4
7	3.8	7.5	8.4	9.2	9.6	9.7
8	2.6	5.5	6.2	7.1	7.4	7.5
9	1.8	4.1	4.7	5.5	5.7	5.8
10	1.3	3.1	3.6	4.2	4.3	4.4
12	0.68	1.6	2.1	2.4	2.6	2.8
14	0.36	0.90	1.3	1.5	1.6	1.7
16	0.19	0.54	0.88	0.96	1.0	1.0
			75 kV$_p$			
0	100	100	100	100	100	100
1	54.0	63.0	68.6	72.4	74.0	74.1
2	34.0	42.0	48.0	50.0	51.6	51.6
3	20.3	29.0	33.4	36.7	38.1	38.3
4	14.0	21.0	24.7	27.9	28.1	28.2
5	9.3	16.0	18.5	21.0	21.9	21.9
6	6.5	11.8	14.0	15.8	16.7	17.2
7	4.4	8.8	10.9	12.6	13.5	13.9
8	3.2	6.5	8.3	10.0	11.2	11.2
9	2.3	5.0	6.4	7.9	8.2	8.8
10	1.7	4.2	5.2	6.3	6.8	6.9
12	0.92	2.4	3.2	4.0	4.5	4.5
14	0.52	1.5	1.9	2.5	2.9	3.0
16	0.29	0.66	1.2	1.6	2.0	2.0

(Harrison RM: Central axis depth-dose data for diagnostic radiology. Phys Med Biol 26:657, 1981)

Table A-5. Percentage Depth Doses: 1.5 mm Al HVT

Depth (cm)	Field Size (cm²)					
	0	7 × 7	10 × 10	15 × 15	20 × 20	30 × 30
			60 kV$_p$			
0	100	100	100	100	100	100
1	64.0	74.2	75.8	77.5	77.8	77.9
2	41.0	53.0	55.0	57.4	57.5	57.6
3	26.5	37.8	40.8	42.0	42.4	43.1
4	17.5	27.3	30.0	31.5	33.2	33.6
5	11.8	20.0	22.5	24.1	24.5	24.7
6	7.9	14.7	16.9	18.4	18.9	19.8
7	5.6	10.9	12.7	14.2	15.0	15.8
8	3.9	8.1	9.6	11.0	11.8	12.6
9	2.9	6.1	7.4	8.6	9.3	10.1
10	2.1	4.6	5.7	6.7	7.5	8.1
12	1.15	2.6	3.5	4.1	4.6	5.4
14	0.66	1.5	2.1	2.5	2.9	3.6
16	0.40	0.86	1.3	1.5	1.8	2.4
			75 kV$_p$			
0	100	100	100	100	100	100
1	64.0	74.2	76.5	78.2	79.3	80.0
2	41.0	53.0	56.0	59.0	59.9	60.6
3	26.5	38.8	41.5	44.9	46.2	47.2
4	18.3	28.3	31.5	34.7	36.0	36.2
5	12.6	21.4	24.0	26.9	28.0	28.7
6	9.0	16.0	18.3	20.9	22.0	22.7
7	6.4	12.1	14.2	16.6	17.8	18.6
8	4.7	9.2	11.0	13.2	14.4	15.2
9	3.4	7.2	8.6	10.5	11.5	12.5
10	2.5	5.6	6.7	8.4	9.1	10.2
12	1.4	3.3	4.0	5.3	6.1	6.9
14	0.83	2.0	2.4	3.4	4.0	4.7
16	0.50	1.2	1.5	2.2	2.6	3.2
			90 kV$_p$			
0	100	100	100	100	100	100
1	64.0	74.2	78.8	79.2	80.1	80.2
2	41.0	53.7	58.4	61.0	61.1	61.2
3	26.5	39.2	43.8	47.0	47.5	48.3
4	18.5	29.7	33.7	36.9	37.8	37.8
5	13.0	22.6	26.0	29.1	30.0	30.7
6	9.5	17.7	20.0	23.0	23.9	25.2
7	6.8	13.2	15.8	18.6	19.7	20.7
8	5.0	10.1	12.5	15.0	16.4	17.0
9	3.7	7.9	9.9	12.2	13.0	14.1
10	2.8	6.3	7.9	10.0	10.6	11.7
12	1.6	3.8	5.0	6.7	7.2	8.2
14	1.0	2.4	3.2	4.5	4.9	5.8
16	0.62	1.5	2.0	3.0	3.3	4.1

(Harrison RM: Central axis depth-dose data for diagnostic radiology. Phys Med Biol 26:657, 1981)

Table A-6. Percentage Depth Doses: 2 mm Al HVT

Depth (cm)	Field Size (cm²) 60 kV$_p$						Field Size (cm²) 75 kV$_p$					
	0	7 × 7	10 × 10	15 × 15	20 × 20	30 × 30	0	7 × 7	10 × 10	15 × 15	20 × 20	30 × 30
0	100	100	100	100	100	100	100	100	100	100	100	100
1	68.0	80.0	83.2	84.0	84.8	84.9	68.0	80.0	83.2	84.0	84.8	84.9
2	45.5	60.8	64.3	66.4	67.1	67.8	45.5	60.8	64.3	66.4	67.1	67.8
3	31.0	46.0	49.8	51.6	52.0	52.3	31.5	46.0	49.8	52.5	53.0	54.3
4	21.0	33.2	38.5	40.0	41.2	41.4	22.0	34.8	38.5	41.0	42.8	43.3
5	14.3	24.8	28.7	31.1	31.7	32.5	15.7	26.5	29.4	32.3	33.6	34.7
6	10.0	18.4	22.0	24.2	25.0	25.6	11.2	20.0	23.1	25.5	27.1	27.8
7	7.2	13.8	16.8	18.8	19.9	20.4	8.2	15.3	18.0	20.4	21.8	22.7
8	5.1	10.4	12.8	14.6	15.8	16.3	5.9	11.8	14.1	16.3	17.4	18.6
9	3.7	7.9	10.1	11.5	12.5	13.1	4.4	9.3	11.0	13.1	14.4	15.4
10	2.7	6.0	7.9	9.1	10.0	10.6	3.3	7.0	8.6	10.5	11.4	12.7
12	1.5	3.5	4.7	5.7	6.3	7.1	1.9	4.3	5.3	6.8	7.2	8.8
14	0.87	2.0	2.8	3.6	4.1	4.7	1.2	2.6	3.3	4.4	5.1	6.1
16	0.51	1.2	1.7	2.3	2.7	3.1	0.70	1.6	2.1	2.8	3.6	4.2

	90 kVp						100 kVp					
	100	100	100	100	100	100	100	100	100	100	100	100
0	100	100	100	100	100	100	100	100	100	100	100	100
1	68.0	80.0	83.2	84.0	84.8	84.9	68.0	80.0	83.2	84.0	84.8	84.9
2	45.5	60.8	64.3	66.4	67.1	67.8	45.5	60.8	64.3	66.4	67.1	67.8
3	31.5	46.0	49.8	52.8	53.8	54.4	31.5	46.0	49.8	52.8	54.2	55.0
4	22.0	35.2	38.5	42.0	43.2	44.3	22.0	35.2	38.5	42.9	44.0	45.0
5	15.7	27.0	31.0	34.0	34.8	36.5	16.0	27.4	31.1	34.8	36.1	37.5
6	11.2	20.9	24.5	27.5	28.2	30.0	11.4	21.7	24.5	28.2	29.7	31.2
7	8.2	16.2	19.5	22.2	23.2	25.1	8.5	16.8	19.8	23.0	24.6	26.1
8	5.9	12.6	15.5	18.0	19.2	21.0	6.3	13.0	16.0	18.8	20.4	21.9
9	4.4	9.8	12.5	14.7	15.7	17.4	4.7	10.5	13.0	15.5	16.5	18.5
10	3.3	7.6	10.1	12.0	12.7	14.5	3.5	8.3	10.5	12.7	13.8	15.7
12	1.9	4.8	6.4	8.0	8.8	10.3	2.0	5.3	6.9	8.6	9.5	11.3
14	1.2	3.0	4.1	5.4	6.0	7.3	1.2	3.4	4.5	5.8	6.8	8.2
16	0.70	1.9	2.6	3.6	4.1	5.2	0.78	2.2	2.9	3.9	4.9	6.0

(Harrison RM: Central axis depth-dose data for diagnostic radiology. Phys Med Biol 26:657, 1981)

Table A-7. Percentage Depth Doses: 3 mm Al HVT

Depth (cm)	Field Size (cm²)					
	0	7 × 7	10 × 10	15 × 15	20 × 20	30 × 30
			75 kV$_p$			
0	100	100	100	100	100	100
1	73.5	87.7	90.4	91.8	92.1	92.5
2	52.0	70.7	74.2	76.0	77.0	77.7
3	37.0	55.2	59.5	62.7	63.7	64.6
4	27.0	43.0	46.4	51.2	52.6	53.0
5	19.0	33.5	37.5	41.4	43.8	44.0
6	14.0	26.4	30.3	33.4	35.7	36.6
7	10.0	20.7	24.0	26.9	29.0	30.1
8	7.5	16.0	19.0	21.6	23.0	24.8
9	5.6	12.4	15.1	17.6	19.0	20.7
10	4.2	9.8	12.0	14.3	15.4	17.2
12	2.5	6.1	7.7	9.4	10.4	12.0
14	1.5	3.8	4.9	6.1	6.9	8.4
16	0.93	2.3	3.1	4.3	4.5	5.9
			90 kV$_p$			
0	100	100	100	100	100	100
1	73.5	87.7	90.4	91.8	92.1	92.5
2	52.0	70.7	74.2	76.0	77.0	77.7
3	37.0	55.2	59.5	62.7	63.7	64.6
4	27.5	43.0	47.4	51.2	52.6	53.7
5	20.0	34.0	38.1	42.2	44.0	44.8
6	14.5	26.6	30.7	34.7	35.7	37.4
7	11.0	20.9	24.5	28.3	29.5	31.5
8	8.1	16.5	19.6	23.0	24.3	26.6
9	6.2	13.0	15.7	19.0	20.1	22.3
10	4.7	10.2	12.6	15.5	16.5	18.7
12	2.8	6.5	8.3	10.5	11.5	13.5
14	1.7	4.1	5.5	7.1	8.2	9.7
16	1.1	2.6	3.6	5.3	5.8	7.0
			100 kV$_p$			
0	100	100	100	100	100	100
1	73.5	87.7	90.4	91.8	92.1	92.5
2	52.0	70.7	74.2	76.0	77.0	77.7
3	37.0	55.2	59.5	62.7	63.7	64.6
4	27.5	43.0	48.0	52.0	52.6	55.0
5	20.5	34.5	38.9	43.0	44.2	46.3
6	15.2	27.0	31.6	35.6	37.1	39.0
7	11.3	21.7	25.5	29.4	31.0	33.0
8	8.7	17.4	20.5	24.3	25.7	28.0
9	6.7	13.7	16.8	20.1	21.5	23.9
10	5.0	10.9	13.7	16.7	17.8	20.4
12	3.1	7.0	9.0	11.6	12.5	14.8
14	1.9	4.5	5.9	8.0	8.8	10.7
16	1.2	2.9	3.9	5.5	6.2	7.7

(Harrison RM: Central axis depth-dose data for diagnostic radiology. Phys Med Biol 26:657, 1981)

Table A-8.   *Percentage Depth Doses: 4 mm Al HVT*

Depth (cm)	Field Size (cm²)					
	0	*7 × 7*	*10 × 10*	*15 × 15*	*20 × 20*	*30 × 30*
			100 kV$_p$			
0	100	100	100	100	100	100
1	76.0	90.6	93.6	94.2	95.0	96.8
2	55.0	75.0	80.2	81.3	83.6	86.0
3	40.5	60.6	66.4	69.5	72.9	73.4
4	30.5	48.5	54.3	58.4	60.5	63.2
5	23.0	38.5	44.5	48.9	51.7	53.9
6	17.0	30.8	36.5	41.0	43.6	46.0
7	13.0	25.2	29.8	34.1	36.6	39.1
8	10.1	20.5	24.3	28.4	30.5	33.2
9	7.7	16.3	19.9	23.7	26.0	28.6
10	5.7	13.1	16.3	19.8	21.6	24.7
12	3.5	8.4	10.8	13.9	15.2	17.9
14	2.2	5.3	7.2	9.7	10.6	13.0
16	1.4	3.4	4.8	6.8	7.2	9.4

(Harrison RM: Central axis depth-dose data for diagnostic radiology. Phys Med Biol 26:657, 1981)

1. All measurements are along central axis of x-ray beam.
2. All measurements are made in water tank.
3. Distance from x-ray source to surface of water tank is 60 cm for Tables A-4 to A-8, and 76 cm for Figures A-7 and A-8.
4. Waveform is not applicable in the case of Harrison's data (Tables A-4 to A-8). Applies to single-phase or three-phase systems as specified in Figures A-7 and A-8 for Kelley and Trout's data.
5. Measurements are probably accurate to within 10%.

To use this technique, the following data are required for each exposure:

1. kVp
2. HVL
3. Source exit distance
4. Patient AP thickness over conceptus
5. Depth of conceptus
6. Field size at entrance skin surface
7. Entrance dose at skin surface over conceptus for radiographic techniques used in examination

Dose to a conceptus is given by the following:

$$D^{(H)} = Q \cdot \frac{P}{100} \cdot \left\{ \left(\frac{S - L}{S - L + d}\right)^2 \cdot \left(1 + \frac{d}{60 \text{ cm}}\right)^2 \right\} \qquad (A\text{-}3)$$

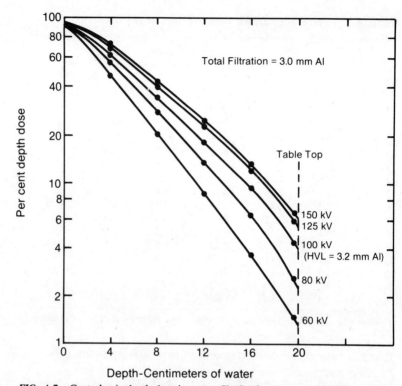

FIG. A-7. Central axis depth dose in water: Single-phase system, 30-inch source to skin distance, 14- × 17-inch field at 40 inches. (Kelley JP, Trout ED: Physical characteristics of radiation from 2-pulse, 12-pulse and 1,000-pulse x-ray equipment. Radiology 100:653, 1971)

$$D^{(KT)} = Q \cdot \frac{P}{100} \cdot \left\{ \left(\frac{S - L}{S - L + d}\right)^2 \cdot \left(1 + \frac{d}{76 \text{ cm}}\right)^2 \right\} \qquad \text{(A-4)}$$

where

- $D^{(H)}$ is the depth dose using data of Tables A-4 to A-8.
- $D^{(KT)}$ is the depth dose using data of Figures A-7 and A-8.
- Q is the surface entrance dose for the study.
- P is the percentage depth dose for the conceptus at depth d.
- S and L are the source exit distance and AP thickness, respectively, as previously defined.

If the free-in-air entrance exposure at the surface of the patient is measured, the equations become

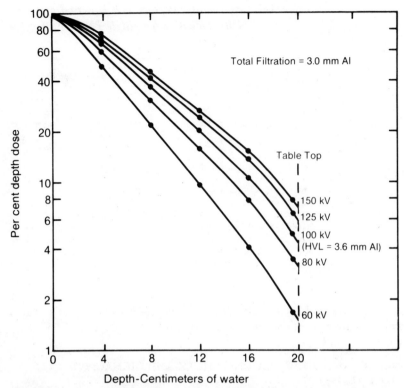

FIG. A-8. Central axis depth dose in water: Three-phase system, 30-inch source to skin distance, 14- × 17-inch field at 40 inches. (Kelley JP, Trout ED: Physical characteristics of radiation from 2-pulse, 12-pulse and 1,000-pulse x-ray equipment. Radiology 100:653, 1971)

$$D^{(H)} = X \cdot f \cdot B \cdot \frac{P}{100} \cdot \left\{ (\frac{S - L}{S - L + d})^2 \cdot (1 + \frac{d}{60 \ cm})^2 \right\} \quad (A\text{-}5)$$

$$D^{(KT)} = X \cdot f \cdot B \cdot \frac{P}{100} \cdot \left\{ (\frac{S - L}{S - L + d})^2 \cdot \ (1 + \frac{d}{76 \ cm})^2 \right\} \quad (A\text{-}6)$$

where

- f   is a factor that converts exposure in roentgen to dose in rad (f = 0.89 rad/R).
- B   is the backscatter factor (Table A-9) that accounts for radiation scattered back to the surface once the beam enters the body.

An advantage of this technique is that it allows for easy interpolation of

Table A-9. **Backscatter Factors as a Function of Peak Tube Potential for Single-Phase, Full-Wave Rectification**

kV	HVL (mm Al)	Backscatter Factor Field size (cm)	
		20 × 25	*35 × 43*
40	1.4	1.16	1.16
60	2.0	1.27	1.27
80	2.7	1.34	1.35
100	3.4	1.38	1.40
130	4.4	1.41	1.45
150	4.9	1.42	1.46

(Trout ED, Kelley JP, Lucas AC: The effect of kilovoltage and filtration on depth-dose. In Janower ML [ed]: Technological Needs for Reduction of Patient Dosage from Diagnostic Radiology, 1963, Courtesy of Charles C. Thomas, Publisher, Springfield, Illinois)

numerous HVL's and kVp's. The disadvantage of this technique is that it requires measurement of entrance dose or the use of backscatter data.

TISSUE–AIR RATIO TECHNIQUE (SCHULZ AND GIGNAC, 1976; SABEL ET AL, 1980)

Tissue–air ratios for converting free-in-air exposure in roentgen at the point in space occupied by the conceptus to dose in rad for the conceptus located at depth d in the patient are given in Tables A-10 through A-17. Figure A-9 provides factors to convert data of Tables A-10 and A-11 from a 40- × 40-cm field to other field sizes. The constraints under which these data were collected include

1. All measurements were along central axis of x-ray beam.
2. All measurements were made in water tank.
3. Distance from x-ray source to point of measurement was 80 cm (Tables A-10 and A-11) and 75 cm (Tables A-12 through A-17).
4. Simulated three-phase ($\pm$ 15% ripple) waveform (Tables A-10 and A-11) and three-phase, six-pulse (Tables A-12 through A-17)
5. Tube current was less than 6 mA for data of Tables A-10 and A-11.

This technique requires that the following data be collected for each radiograph:

1. kVp
2. HVL

Table A-10. *Tissue–Air Ratios (rad/R) for 40-*
× 40-cm Field and Total Filtration
of 2.5 mm Al

Depth (cm)	70	80	kV 90	100	120
0	1.02	1.09	1.12	1.14	1.15
2	1.00	1.07	1.10	1.13	1.15
4	0.709	0.794	0.834	0.878	1.00
6	0.501	0.580	0.621	0.665	0.742
8	0.354	0.423	0.463	0.504	0.573
10	0.250	0.309	0.345	0.382	0.443
12	0.177	0.226	0.257	0.289	0.342
14	0.125	0.165	0.192	0.219	0.264
16	0.088	0.120	0.143	0.166	0.204
18	0.062	0.088	0.107	0.126	0.158
20	0.044	0.064	0.080	0.095	0.122

(Schulz RJ, Gignac C: Application of tissue–air ratios for patient doses in diagnostic radiology. Radiology 120:687, 1976)

3. Depth of conceptus
4. Central-axis free-in-air exposure at level of conceptus
5. Field size at level of conceptus

The absorbed dose to the conceptus is given by

$$D^{(SG)} = T \cdot X^* \tag{A-7}$$

$$D^{(S)} = T \cdot X^* \tag{A-8}$$

where

- $D^{(SG)}$ is the dose acquired using Tables A-10 and A-11.
- $D^{(S)}$ is the dose acquired using the data of Tables A-12 through A-17.
- T is the appropriate tissue–air ratio.
- X^* is the free-in-air exposure at conceptus position.

An advantage of this technique is that it allows for a wide range of HVL's, kVp's, and field sizes.

**PATIENT-SIMULATED NORMALIZED DEPTH-DOSE
ESTIMATES (ROSENSTEIN, 1976)**

Normalized dose to the conceptus in units of rad per 1-R free-in-air entrance exposure are given in Table A-18. The conditions under which these data were accumulated include

Table A-11. Tissue–Air Ratios (rad/R) for 40- × 40-cm Field and Total Filtration of 3.5 mm Al

Depth (cm)	70	80	kV 90	100	120
0	1.07	1.10	1.12	1.14	1.15
2	1.06	1.09	1.11	1.15	1.20
4	0.791	0.845	0.904	0.955	1.09
6	0.566	0.625	0.679	0.726	0.813
8	0.406	0.461	0.510	0.552	0.630
10	0.291	0.340	0.383	0.420	0.489
12	0.208	0.250	0.288	0.320	0.379
14	0.149	0.185	0.217	0.243	0.294
16	0.107	0.136	0.163	0.185	0.228
18	0.077	0.100	0.122	0.141	0.177
20	0.055	0.074	0.092	0.107	0.137

(Schulz RJ, Gignac C: Application of tissue–air ratios for patient doses in diagnostic radiology. Radiology 120:687, 1976)

Table A-12. Tissue–Air Ratios (rad/R) for Total Filtration of 2.6 mm Al and HVL of 2.2 mm Al at 60 kVp

Depth (cm)	Field Size (cm²) 10 × 10	15 × 15	20 × 20	30 × 30
0	1.11	1.12	1.12	1.12
1	0.980	1.02	1.02	1.05
2	0.802	0.840	0.844	0.859
3	0.633	0.668	0.674	0.697
4	0.493	0.535	0.545	0.562
5	0.387	0.429	0.439	0.459
6	0.305	0.344	0.354	0.375
7	0.239	0.276	0.285	0.305
8	0.188	0.221	0.230	0.249
9	0.148	0.178	0.186	0.204
10	0.116	0.142	0.149	0.166
12	0.072	0.092	0.096	0.110
14	0.045	0.059	0.063	0.074
16	0.027	0.038	0.040	0.049
18	0.017	0.025	0.026	0.032
20	0.011	0.016	0.018	0.022

(Sabel M, Bednar W, Weishaar J: Investigation of the exposure to radiation of the embryo/fetus in the course of radiographic examinations during pregnancy. First communication: Tissue–air ratios for x rays with tube voltages between 60 kV and 120 kV. Strahlentherapie 156:502, 1980)

Table A-13.   *Tissue–Air Ratios (rad/R) for Total Filtration of 2.6 mm Al and Half-Value Layer of 2.6 mm Al at 70 kVp*

Depth (cm)	Field Size (cm²)			
	10 × 10	*15 × 15*	*20 × 20*	*30 × 30*
0	1.10	1.14	1.15	1.15
1	1.05	1.09	1.09	1.11
2	0.901	0.928	0.928	0.954
3	0.727	0.766	0.768	0.793
4	0.588	0.622	0.633	0.661
5	0.473	0.511	0.525	0.553
6	0.380	0.420	0.436	0.463
7	0.305	0.345	0.361	0.388
8	0.245	0.284	0.299	0.325
9	0.197	0.233	0.249	0.272
10	0.158	0.191	0.207	0.228
12	0.102	0.129	0.142	0.159
14	0.066	0.087	0.098	0.112
16	0.043	0.059	0.067	0.079
18	0.027	0.039	0.046	0.055
20	0.018	0.027	0.032	0.039

(Sabel M, Bednar W, Weishaar J: Investigation of the exposure to radiation of the embryo/fetus in the course of radiographic examinations during pregnancy. First communication: Tissue–air ratios for x rays with tube voltages between 60 kV and 120 kV. Strahlentherapie 156:502, 1980)

1. Only mathematical calculations were used (Monte-Carlo technique).
2. Data apply to standard radiographic geometry.
3. Data apply only to a "standard"-size patient.
4. Uterus was at 8-cm depth from anterior surface.
5. Distance of x-ray source to patient's surface was 77 cm.

To use this technique, the following data are required for each radiograph:

1. Type of study
2. HVL
3. Free-in-air entrance exposure in roentgen.
4. S, L, and d are required to apply the bracketed inverse square correction.

Using these data, the dose to the conceptus is given by

$$D^{(R)} = X \cdot \delta \cdot \left[\frac{(S - L)^2}{(S - L + d)^2} \cdot (1 + \frac{d}{102 \text{ cm}})^2 \right] \qquad (A\text{-}9)$$

Table A-14. *Tissue–Air Ratios (rad/R) for Total Filtration of 2.6 mm Al and HVL of 3.0 mm Al at 80 kVp*

Depth (cm)	Field Size (cm²)			
	10 × 10	15 × 15	20 × 20	30 × 30
0	1.14	1.19	1.19	1.19
1	1.09	1.15	1.15	1.15
2	0.936	1.03	1.02	1.02
3	0.774	0.870	0.869	0.865
4	0.632	0.722	0.729	0.735
5	0.517	0.597	0.610	0.626
6	0.423	0.494	0.511	0.533
7	0.346	0.408	0.428	0.453
8	0.283	0.338	0.358	0.386
9	0.232	0.279	0.299	0.328
10	0.189	0.231	0.251	0.279
12	0.127	0.158	0.176	0.202
14	0.085	0.108	0.123	0.146
16	0.057	0.074	0.087	0.106
18	0.038	0.051	0.060	0.077
20	0.025	0.034	0.042	0.056

(Sabel M, Bednar W, Weishaar J: Investigation of the exposure to radiation of the embryo/fetus in the course of radiographic examinations during pregnancy. First communication: Tissue–air ratios for x rays with tube voltages between 60 kV and 120 kV. Strahlentherapie 156:502, 1980)

where δ is the appropriate normalized uterine dose estimate. The advantages of this technique are that it takes into account the chemical composition of body tissues, including bone; it has applicability for lateral views; and it is easy to use. The disadvantage of this technique is that it may give erroneous dose estimations for patients differing significantly from the assumed anatomic dimensions. There is also no allowance for field size variations.

EXAMPLE NO. 1

Use each of the previous techniques to estimate conceptus dose for a patient who had an AP supine KUB radiograph. The following data apply:

Peak kilovoltage	= 75 kVp
Waveform	= three-phase
HVL	= 3 mm Al
Filtration	= 3.5 mm Al (from Table A-2)
Output, M (h′ = 1 m)	= 7.2 mR/mAs (from Fig. A-2)

Table A-15.   *Tissue–Air Ratios (rad/R) for Total Filtration of 2.6 mm Al and HVL of 3.5 mm Al at 90 kVp*

Depth (cm)	Field Size (cm^2)			
	10 × 10	*15 × 15*	*20 × 20*	*30 × 30*
0	1.13	1.17	1.20	1.20
1	1.11	1.15	1.18	1.18
2	0.971	1.02	1.06	1.04
3	0.809	0.865	0.910	0.901
4	0.668	0.732	0.776	0.770
5	0.550	0.615	0.659	0.662
6	0.452	0.517	0.560	0.570
7	0.372	0.435	0.476	0.490
8	0.306	0.366	0.404	0.421
9	0.252	0.308	0.343	0.362
10	0.207	0.259	0.291	0.312
12	0.141	0.183	0.211	0.231
14	0.095	0.130	0.152	0.171
16	0.065	0.092	0.109	0.126
18	0.044	0.065	0.079	0.094
20	0.030	0.046	0.057	0.069

(Sabel M, Bednar W, Weishaar J: Investigation of the exposure to radiation of the embryo/fetus in the course of radiographic examinations during pregnancy. First communication: Tissue–air ratios for x rays with tube voltages between 60 kV and 120 kV. Strahlentherapie 156:502, 1980)

Tube current and exposure time	= 50 mAs
Field size	= 36 × 43 cm at film, with long axis parallel to body (film 102 cm from source)
S	= 97 cm
Patient-thickness, L	= 20 cm
S − L	= 77 cm (this is source to patient distance)
Conceptus depth, d	= 6 cm
S − L + d	= 83 cm

Technique no. 1 (normalized depth dose)

Output, M (h = 0.77 m)	= 12 mR/mAs (from Eq. A-1)
Free-in-air entrance exposure, X	= 0.6 R (12 mR/mAs · 50 mAs)
Normalized depth dose, N	= 0.53 rad/R ± 10% (approximated by interpolation from Figs. A-3 and A-4)

Table A-16.   **Tissue–Air Ratios (rad/R) for Total Filtration of 2.6 mm Al and HVL of 3.9 mm Al at 100 kVp**

Depth (cm)	Field Size (cm²)			
	10 × 10	*15 × 15*	*20 × 20*	*30 × 30*
0	1.15	1.20	1.21	1.21
1	1.11	1.18	1.19	1.19
2	0.998	1.09	1.09	1.09
3	0.842	0.928	0.945	0.945
4	0.702	0.794	0.812	0.830
5	0.584	0.674	0.696	0.720
6	0.486	0.572	0.596	0.626
7	0.404	0.486	0.511	0.543
8	0.336	0.412	0.438	0.472
9	0.279	0.350	0.375	0.410
10	0.233	0.298	0.322	0.355
12	0.161	0.214	0.236	0.268
14	0.111	0.154	0.173	0.202
16	0.077	0.111	0.128	0.152
18	0.053	0.081	0.094	0.115
20	0.037	0.058	0.069	0.087

(Sabel M, Bednar W, Weishaar J: Investigation of the exposure to radiation of the embryo/fetus in the course of radiographic examinations during pregnancy. First communication: Tissue–air ratios for x rays with tube voltages between 60 kV and 120 kV. Strahlentherapie 156:502, 1980)

From Equation A-2

$$D^{(RGB)} = 0.53 \text{ rad/R} \cdot 0.6 \text{ R} \cdot \left\{ (\frac{77 \text{ cm}}{83 \text{ cm}})^2 \cdot (1 + \frac{6 \text{ cm}}{102 \text{ cm}})^2 \right\}$$

$$\boxed{D^{(RGB)} = 0.31 \pm 0.03 \text{ rad}}$$

Technique no. 2 (percent depth dose)

Entrance field-size = 27 × 32 cm (calculated from simple geometry of the situation)

Backscatter factor, B = ∼1.35 (from Table A-9)

Free-in-air entrance exposure, X = 0.6 R (see previous technique)

Percentage depth dose, P = 36.6 (from Table A-8, 30- × 30-cm field size); 40.0 (from Fig. A-8)

Table A-17. Tissue–Air Ratios (rad/R) for Total Filtration of 2.6 mm Al and HVL of 4.7 mm Al at 120 kVp

Depth (cm)	Field Size (cm²)			
	10 × 10	15 × 15	20 × 20	30 × 30
0	1.16	1.23	1.23	1.25
1	1.16	1.23	1.23	1.29
2	1.02	1.12	1.12	1.18
3	0.893	1.02	1.02	1.09
4	0.760	0.884	0.893	0.954
5	0.638	0.756	0.781	0.836
6	0.537	0.648	0.677	0.731
7	0.452	0.555	0.588	0.639
8	0.380	0.475	0.510	0.558
9	0.319	0.407	0.443	0.488
10	0.269	0.348	0.384	0.427
12	0.191	0.256	0.289	0.326
14	0.135	0.187	0.218	0.249
16	0.095	0.137	0.164	0.191
18	0.067	0.101	0.123	0.146
20	0.048	0.074	0.093	0.112

(Sabel M, Bednar W, Weishaar J: Investigation of the exposure to radiation of the embryo/fetus in the course of radiographic examinations during pregnancy. First communication: Tissue–air ratios for x rays with tube voltages between 60 kV and 120 kV. Strahlentherapie 156:502, 1980)

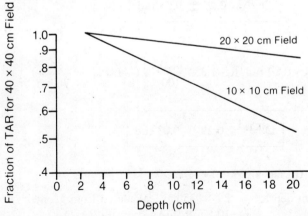

FIG. A-9. Effect of field size on tissue–air ratios. The effect of field size is independent of peak potential from 70 kVp to 120 kVp and for filtration from 2.5 mm to 3.5 mm Al. (Schulz RJ, Gignac C: Application of tissue-air ratios for patient doses in diagnostic radiology. Radiology 120:687, 1976)

Table A-18.   *Conceptus dose (rad) for 1-R entrance skin exposure (free-in-air).*

Conditions	SID = 102 cm (40″)
	Film Size = Field Size = 35.6 × 43.2 cm (14″ × 17″)
Projection	Retrograde pyelogram, KUB, barium enema, lumbosacral spine, IVP, renal arteriogram[a]

Beam Quality HVL (mm Al)	Embryo (Uterus) Dose in rad					
	1.5	*2.0*	*2.5*	*3.0*	*3.5*	*4.0*
AP	0.133	0.199	0.265	0.330	0.392	0.451
PA	0.56	0.90	0.130	0.174	0.222	0.273
Lateral	0.13	0.23	0.37	0.53	0.71	0.91

[a]Similar data apply for pelvic radiography.
(Rosenstein M: Handbook of Selected Organ Doses for Projections Common in Diagnostic Radiology, HEW publication (FDA) 76-8031. Rockville, Maryland, Bureau of Radiological Health, 1976)

From Equation A-5

$$D^{(H)} = 0.6R \cdot 0.89 \text{ rad/R} \cdot 1.35 \cdot \frac{36.6}{100} \cdot \left\{ (\frac{77}{83})^2 \cdot (1 + \frac{6}{60 \text{ cm}})^2 \right\}$$

$$\boxed{D^{(H)} = 0.27 \pm 0.03 \text{ rad}}$$

From Equation A-6

$$D^{(KT)} = 0.6 \text{ R} \cdot 0.89 \text{ rad/R} \cdot 1.35 \cdot \frac{40.0}{100} \cdot \left\{ (\frac{77}{83})^2 \cdot (1 + \frac{6}{76 \text{ cm}})^2 \right\}$$

$$\boxed{D^{(KT)} = 0.29 + 0.03 \text{ rad}}$$

Technique no. 3 (tissue–air ratio)

Field size at 6-cm depth	= 29 × 35 cm (calculated from geometry)
M (h = 0.83 m)	= 10.5 mR/mAs (from Eq. A-1)
X*	= 0.52 R (10.5 mR/mAs × 50 mAs)
$T^{(SG)}$	= ∼0.60 rad/R (estimated from Table A-11)
$T^{(S)}$	= ∼0.53 rad/R (estimated from Table A-14)

From Equation A-7

$$D^{(SG)} = 0.60 \text{ rad}/R \cdot 0.52 \text{ R}$$

$$\boxed{D^{(SG)} = 0.31 \pm 0.03 \text{ rad}}$$

From Equation A-8

$$D^{(S)} = 0.53 \text{ rad}/R \cdot 0.52 \text{ R}$$

$$\boxed{D^{(S)} = 0.28 \pm 0.03 \text{ rad}}$$

Technique no. 4 (Patient-simulated normalized dose estimate)

Free-in-air entrance exposure　　= 0.6 R (see Technique No. 1, Example No. 1)

Normalized dose, δ (AP view)　= 0.330 rad/R (from Table A-18)

From Equation A-9

$$D^{(R)} = 0.6 \text{ R} \cdot 0.330 \text{ rad} \cdot \left\{ \left(\frac{77 \text{ cm}}{83 \text{ cm}}\right)^2 \cdot \left(1 + \frac{6 \text{ cm}}{77 \text{ cm}}\right)^2 \right\}$$

$$\boxed{D^{(R)} = 0.20 \text{ rad}}$$

This estimate is about two thirds the estimate of the previous techniques. The error is the value of δ and is due to the difference in conceptus depth, which is actually 6 cm but is assumed to be 8 cm by Rosenstein. Harrison's data (Table A-7) can be used to show that 2 cm of tissue will reduce the beam intensity by about 32%. The calculation from Rosenstein can be appropriately corrected by assuming the calculated dose is only 68% of the actual dose. This caveat should be remembered when applying Rosenstein's data to conceptus dose calculations. In this example, the difference is of no consequence. In cases of high doses delivered to a severely anteverted or retroverted uterus, it can make a consequential difference. The corrected dose in this case is

$$\boxed{D^{(R)} \text{ (corrected)} = \frac{0.20 \text{ rad}}{0.68} = 0.29 \text{ rad}}$$

EXAMPLE No. 2:

Estimate the fluoroscopic dose to the conceptus of the same patient who also received direct PA fluoroscopy to the uterus. The relevant data are

Peak kilovoltage	= 110 kVp
Waveform	= three-phase
HVL	= 4 mm Al
Tube current and exposure time	= 2 mA for 1 min = 2 mA · min
Filtration	= ~3 mm Al (from Table A-2)
Output, M (h′ = 0.38 m)	= 3.8 R/mA · min (from Table A-3)
Field size at exit side of patient	= 23-cm diameter (diameter of image intensifier)
S	= 60 cm
Patient-thickness, L	= 20 cm
S − L	= 40 cm (this is source to patient distance)
Conceptus PA depth, d	= 14 cm
S − L + d	= 54 cm

Technique no. 1 (normalized depth dose)

Output M (h = 0.40 m)	= 3.4 R/(mA · min) (from Eq. A-1)
Free-in-air entrance exposure, X	= 6.8 R [3.4 R/(mA · min) × 2mA· min]
Normalized depth dose, N	= 0.15 rad/R (Figs. A-3 and A-4)

From Equation A-2

$$D^{(RGB)} = 0.15 \text{ rad/R} \cdot 6.8 \text{ R} \cdot \left\{ (\frac{40 \text{ cm}}{54 \text{ cm}})^2 \cdot (1 + \frac{14 \text{ cm}}{102 \text{ cm}})^2 \right\}$$

$$\boxed{D^{(RGB)} = 0.72 \pm 0.07 \text{ rad}}$$

Technique No. 2 (Percent depth dose)

Entrance field-size	= 15-cm diameter (calculated from geometry)
Backscatter factor, B	= 1.38 (from Table A-9)
Free-in-air entrance exposure, X	= 6.8 R (see previous technique)
Percentage depth dose, P	= 9.7% (from Table A-8); 15% (from Fig. A-8)

From Equation A-5

$$D^{(H)} = 6.8 \text{ R} \cdot 0.89 \text{ rad/R} \cdot 1.38 \cdot \frac{9.7}{100} \cdot \left\{ \left(\frac{40 \text{ cm}}{54 \text{ cm}}\right)^2 \cdot \quad (1 + \frac{14 \text{ cm}}{60 \text{ cm}})^2 \right\}$$

$$\boxed{D^{(H)} = 0.68 \pm 0.07 \text{ rad}}$$

From Equation A-6

$$D^{(KT)} = 6.8 \text{ R} \cdot 0.89 \text{ rad/R} \cdot 1.38 \cdot \frac{15}{100} \cdot \left[\left(\frac{40}{54}\right)^2 \cdot (1 + \frac{14 \text{ cm}}{76 \text{ cm}})^2 \right]$$

$$\boxed{D^{(KT)} = 0.97 \text{ rad}}$$

Note that this is considerably higher than the $D^{(H)}$ estimate of 0.68 rad. This is due to the fact that the data of Figure A-8 apply only to an entrance field size of 27 $\times$ 32 cm, whereas the actual field size is only 15 cm in diameter. Harrison's data (Table A-8) indicate that at 14-cm depth the percent depth dose for a 15- $\times$ 15-cm field is about 75% that of a 30- $\times$ 30-cm field. Using this factor to correct $D^{(KT)}$ we get

$$\boxed{D^{(KT)} \text{ (corrected)} = 0.73 \pm 0.07 \text{ rad}}$$

Technique No. 3 (Tissue–air ratio)

Field size at 14-cm depth = 21-cm diameter (calculated from geometry)

Field size correction factor for tissue–air ratio of Table A-11 = 0.88

Output, M (h = 0.54 m) = 1.9 R/mA min (from Eq. A-1)

X* = 3.8 R (1.9 R/mA min $\times$ 2 mA min)

$T^{(SG)}$ (uncorrected for field size) = 0.25 rad/R (estimated from Tables A-10 and A-11)

$T^{(SG)}$ (corrected for field size) = 0.22 rad/R (0.25 rad/R $\times$ 0.8)

$T^{(S)}$ = 0.19 rad/R (estimated from Table A-16)

From Equation A-7

$$D^{(SG)} = 0.22 \text{ rad}/R \cdot 3.8 \text{ R}$$

$$\boxed{D^{(SG)} = 0.84 \pm 0.08 \text{ rad}}$$

From Equation A-8

$$D^{(S)} = 0.19 \text{ rad}/R \cdot 3.8 \text{ R}$$

$$\boxed{D^{(S)} = 0.72 \pm 0.07 \text{ rad}}$$

Technique No. 4 (Patient-simulated normalized dose)

Free-in-air entrance exposure, X   = 6.8 R (see Technique No. 1,
                                                    Example No. 2)
Normalized dose, δ (PA view)   = 0.273 rad/R (from Table A-18)

From Equation A-9

$$D^{(R)} = 6.8 \text{ R} \cdot 0.273 \text{ rad}/R \cdot \left\{ \left(\frac{40}{54}\right)^2 \cdot \left(1 + \frac{14}{77}\right)^2 \right\}$$

$$D^{(R)} = 1.4 \text{ rad}$$

Note that this estimate is considerably higher than the previous ones because this model assumes the conceptus to be 12-cm deep, with an entrance field of 30 × 36 cm. Using Table A-8, the 12-cm percent depth dose for a 30 × 30-cm field is 17.9%. For a 15 × 15-cm field, the 14-cm percent depth dose is 9.7%. Using these figures to correct $D^{(R)}$ we get

$$\boxed{D^{(R)} \text{ (corrected)} = 0.77 \text{ rad}}$$

Note in this case that $D^{(R)}$ (uncorrected) was about a factor of 2 too high. Care must be exercised when applying this data.

Notes on Uncertainties

When corrected for conceptus depth and field size, all four techniques yield reasonable dose estimates. The differences in calculated doses among the techniques are attributable to the differences in the way the measurements were made and in the material composition and shape of the phantoms used as well as in the estimation of the backscatter factor. Nevertheless, the differences are small compared to the errors incurred from uncertainty in the actual conceptus depth. Even if measured by ultrasound with a partially filled bladder, the position is still uncertain by about 2 cm because of movement of the uterus under the force of gravity and with bladder expansion. Harrison's depth-dose data (Table A-7) indicate that a $\pm$ 2-cm uncertainty means the calculation may be 31% too low or 48% too high. A reasonable range of conceptus dose in Example No. 1 is therefore from 0.2 rad to 0.4 rad for the radiographic example. Unless the uterine depth is more accurately established, conceptus dose cannot be more accurately determined.

A similar circumstance is applicable to the fluoroscopic example. Harrison's data (Table A-8) indicate that a $\pm$ 2-cm uncertainty in conceptus depth means the calculations may be 30% too low or 43% too high. The dose range for this example is from 0.5 rad to 1.0 rad.

There are additional practical uncertainties such as the fluoroscopic duration of direct exposure to the conceptus. This and others are reviewed in Chapter 9 and should be incorporated into the dose-range estimate.

Out-of-Field Dose Calculations for Wide Field-of-View Radiography

When the conceptus is outside the field-of-view of the radiograph, dose will depend on how far the conceptus is from the edge of the radiographic field. Figure A-10 is a plot of conceptus dose expressed as a percent of the entrance dose. It is a function of depth and distance from the edge of the radiographic field and is estimated from depth-dose data of Trout and associates (1963). The dose drops off rapidly at the edge of the field. The estimated dose is given by

$$D = Q \cdot p$$

or

$$D = B \cdot f \cdot X \cdot p \qquad \text{(A-10)}$$

where p is the out-of-field percent depth dose, and f, X, B, and Q are previously defined.

EXAMPLE NO. 3

Assuming the same techniques as in Example No. 1, we consider the case where a conceptus is at least 3 cm from the dark edge of the radiographic field. From Figure A-10, a conservative estimate of the dose is 9% that of the entrance dose.

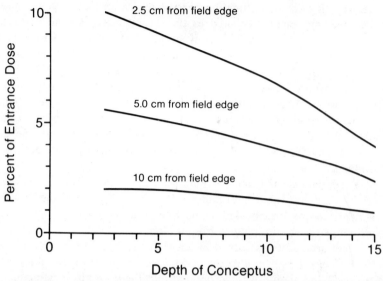

FIG. A-10. Conceptus dose from scatter radiation expressed as the function of percent of the entrance dose for various conceptus depths and distances of radiographic field from conceptus. (Adapted from Trout ED, Kelley JP, Lucas AC: The effect of kilovoltage and filtration on depth–dose. In Janower ML (ed): Technological Needs for Reduction of Patient Dosage from Diagnostic Radiology, Springfield, Illinois, Charles C Thomas, 1963)

Equation A-10 yields

$$D = 1.35 \cdot 0.89 \ \text{rad}/R \cdot 0.6 \ R \cdot 0.09$$

$$\boxed{D = 0.065 \ \text{rad}}$$

If the conceptus is judged to be more than 10 cm from the edge of the field, a rule of thumb is that the conceptus's dose is less than 2% of the entrance dose.

EXAMPLE NO. 4

Use the same data as in Example No. 1, but assume the conceptus is 10 cm from the edge of the field. The dose would be

$$D = 1.35 \cdot 0.89 \ \text{rad}/R \cdot 0.6 \ R \cdot 0.02$$

$$\boxed{D = 0.014 \ \text{rad}}$$

For examinations where the conceptus is 25 cm or more from the edge of the field (outside the abdomen), the dose is so small that it can be considered negligible unless an extraordinary number of radiographs are acquired. In this case we recommend using the tables of Rosenstein (1976) to roughly estimate the dose.

In-Field Dose Calculations for Computed Tomography

Although there is considerable literature on the topic of doses from computed tomography (CT), there is only a sparse amount of literature relevant to applications in pregnant patients. Using plastic cylinders 32 cm in diameter and 16 cm in diameter, Shope and co-workers (1982) measured surface dose and central-axis dose from a variety of CT machines. They also measured the dose for multiple-slice scans. Although the multiple-slice scans increase the surface dose by a factor of 1.2 to 2 over that from a single-slice scan, the dose at the center may be increased by a factor of 3 to 5. The dose to the uterus of a patient in early pregnancy should be greater than the central-axis dose and less than the surface dose for scans that image the pregnancy. From the data of Shope and co-workers, we estimate that the uterine dose ranges from about 40% to 100% of the surface dose for a multiple-slice study. Dose to a conceptus from CT is, therefore, approximately 70% ± 30% of the maximum surface dose.

McCullough and Payne (1978) tabulate maximum surface doses to a simulated body phantom for a number of radiographic conditions from several CT scanners. Depending on the scanner and the radiographic technique employed in the scans, surface doses from a multiple-slice scan can range anywhere from about 1.2 rad to about 15 rad. Conceptus dose would therefore range anywhere from about 0.5 rad to 15 rad for direct CT exposure.

EXAMPLE NO. 5

A patient received a pelvic CT study that included 15 consecutive slices. The conceptus was visible on three of the slices. Calculate conceptus dose if the maximum multiple-slice surface dose was 4.5 rad.

The dose is 70% ± 30% of 4.5 rad.

D (lowest estimate)   = 0.4 · 4.5 rad = 1.8 rad
D (median estimate)   = 0.7 · 4.5 rad = 3.2 rad
D (maximum estimate)   = 4.5 rad

A more accurate estimate can be made by direct measurement under simulated conditions.

Out-of-Field Dose Calculations for Computed Tomography

The dose to a conceptus from scatter and leakage radiation may be estimated from the data of Bassano and associates (1977). They list the scatter-radiation dose to male testes from multiple-slice scans of a delta-scan 50 machine. This is a 180° scanner and, for their techniques, the maximum surface dose from a multiple-slice scan was approximately 1.5 rad. By symmetry from their Figure 8, we estimate that the surface dose from an equivalent 360° scan would have been approximately 2 rad. In Figure A-11, we plot an approximation of the fractional uterine dose as a function of distance from the primary scan site.

EXAMPLE NO. 6:

A patient received 20 single-slice scans at 1-cm intervals across the liver. The most inferior scan was judged to be 6 cm from the conceptus. The multiple-slice surface dose was 4.5 rad. The scanner uses a 360° rotation. Estimate the conceptus dose.

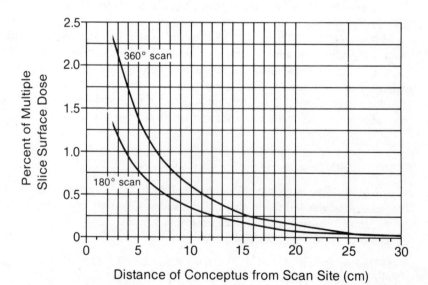

FIG. A-11. Percent conceptus dose from extrauterine CT scans. (Adapted from Bassano DA, Chamberlain CC, Mozley JM et al: Physical performance and dosemetric characteristics of the Δ-scan 50 whole body/brain scanner. Radiology 123:455, 1977)

From Figure A-11, the liver-scan dose to the uterus expressed as a percent of the multiple-slice surface dose is tabulated below for each slice as a function of distance from the uterus:

6 cm	1.2%	11 cm	0.5%	16 cm	0.3%	21 cm	0.2%
7 cm	1.0%	12 cm	0.5%	17 cm	0.2%	22 cm	0.2%
8 cm	0.8%	13 cm	0.4%	18 cm	0.2%	23 cm	0.1%
9 cm	0.7%	14 cm	0.3%	19 cm	0.2%	24 cm	0.1%
10 cm	0.6%	15 cm	0.3%	20 cm	0.2%	25 cm	0.1%

Sum of all 20 slices = 8.1%

Adding up contributions from each slice, we estimate that the dose to the uterus is

$$D = 0.081 \cdot 4.5 \text{ rad} \approx 0.4 \text{ rad}$$

Our experience indicates that this estimate may be too low by a factor of 2, depending on conceptus depth. The most reasonable estimate of conceptus dose is between 0.4 rad and 0.8 rad.

References

Bassano DA, Chamberlain CC, Mozley JM et al: Physical performance, and dosimetric characteristics of the Δ-scan 50 whole body/brain scanner. Radiology 123:455, 1977

Gray JE, Winkler NT, Stears J et al: Quality Control in Diagnostic Imaging, pp 90–94. Baltimore, Maryland, University Park Press, 1983

Hale J: The homogeneity factor for pulsating potential x-ray beams in the diagnostic energy region. Radiology 86:147, 1966

Harrison RM: Central axis depth-dose data for diagnostic radiology. Phys Med Biol 26:657, 1981

Johns HE, Cunningham JR: The Physics of Radiology. Springfield, Illinois, Charles C. Thomas, 1969

Kelley JP, Trout ED: Physical Characteristics of the Radiation from 2-pulse, 12-pulse, and 1000-pulse x-ray equipment. Radiology 100:653, 1971

McCullough EC, Cameron JR: Exposure rates from diagnostic x-ray units. Br J Radiol 43:448, 1970

McCullough EC, Payne TJ: Patient dosage in computed tomography. Radiology 129:457, 1978

National Council on Radiation Protection and Measurements (NCRP): Medical X-ray and Gamma-ray Protection for Energies up to 10 MeV, report No. 33. Washington, DC, NCRP, 1968

National Council on Radiation Protection and Measurements (NCRP): Medical Radiation Exposure of Pregnant and Potentially Pregnant Women, report No. 54. Washington, DC, NCRP, 1977

Ragozzino MW, Gray JE, Burke TM et al: Estimation and minimization of fetal absorbed dose: Data from common radiographic examinations. AJR, 137:667, 1981

Rosenstein M: Organ Doses in Diagnostic Radiology, HEW publication (FDA) 76-8030. Rockville, Maryland, Bureau of Radiological Health, 1976a.

Rosenstein M: Handbook of Selected Organ Doses for Projections Common in Diagnostic Radiology, HEW publication (FDA) 76-8031. Rockville, Maryland, Bureau of Radiological Health, 1976b

Sabel M, Bednar W, Wieshaar J: Investigation of the exposure to radiation of the embryo/fetus in the course of radiographic examinations during pregnancy. First communication: Tissue–air ratios for x-rays with tube voltages between 60 kV and 120 kV. Strahlentherapie 156:502, 1980

Schulz RJ, Gignac C: Application of tissue–air ratios for patient dosage in diagnostic radiology. Radiology 120:687, 1976

Shope TB, Morgan TJ, Showalter CK: Radiation dosimetry survey of computed tomography systems from ten manufacturers. Br J Radiol 55:60, 1982

Trout ED, Kelley JP: Leakage radiation through lead glass fluoroscopic screen assemblies. Radiology 82:977, 1964

Trout ED, Kelley JP, Lucas AC: The effect of kilovoltage and filtration on depth-dose. In Janower ML (ed): Technological Needs for Reduction of Patient Dosage from Diagnostic Radiology. Springfield, Illinois, Charles C. Thomas, 1963

Appendix B
Conceptus Dose Calculations for Radionuclide Studies

The dose to a conceptus from a radiopharmaceutical concentrated within the conceptus or within an organ of the pregnant patient is given by (Loevinger and Berman, 1976):

$$D(c \leftarrow s) = \tilde{A}_s \cdot \frac{\sum_i \Delta_i \phi_i(c \leftarrow s)}{m_c} \tag{B-1}$$

- $D(c \leftarrow s)$ is the dose to the conceptus, c, resulting from radiation emanating from the source organ, s.
- $\tilde{A}_s$ is the number of radionuclide disintegrations, integrated over all time, that occur in the source organ. This is conventionally called the *cumulated activity in organ s* and is usually expressed in units of (μCi $\cdot$ hr) or (Bq $\cdot$ s).
- Δ_i is the mean energy emitted for each radiative emission of a single radionuclide (Dillman and Von der Lage, 1975).
- $\phi_i(c \leftarrow s)$ is the average fraction of Δ_i absorbed by the conceptus (Snyder et al, 1978; Ellett and Humes, 1971).
- $\sum_i$ means that the product $\Delta_i \phi_i$ (c $\leftarrow$ s) is summed over all radiative emissions of the radionuclide.
- m_c is the mass of the conceptus (Gillespie, 1950; Kereiakes and Rosenstein, 1980, Table 14).

$\tilde{A}_s$ depends on how the radioactivity within the organ changes with time. This, in turn, depends on the uptake and elimination of the radiopharmaceutical from the organ as well as the physical decay of the radionuclide. A plot of radioactivity within the organ versus time might take the form of a continual rise from zero, a leveling off to a maximum, and a continual decline afterwards. On the other hand, radioactivity may periodically rise and fall, such as with radiopharmaceuticals accumulating in the bladder and then being intermittently eliminated. Whatever the form, if we know the radioactivity within the organ as a function of time, integration over all time yields $\tilde{A}_s$. This is mathematically expressed as

$$\tilde{A}_s = \int_0^\infty A_s(t)\, dt \qquad (B\text{-}2)$$

where $A_s(t)$ describes the time dependence of the radioactivity in organ s.

It is not practical to think that $A_s(t)$ could be determined for each individual patient and source organ. Approximations based on experience in a number of other patients are necessary. A limited amount of data on $A_s(t)$ and $\tilde{A}_s$ are available. (Kereiakes and Rosenstein, 1980, Table 7; MIRD Committee, 1975, 1976; Berman, 1977; Lathrop et al, 1972).

A sometimes useful estimation of $\tilde{A}_s$ can be performed if the activity is rapidly taken up by the organ and is less rapidly released in a functional form approaching an exponential. In this event

$$\tilde{A}_s = F \cdot A_T \int_0^\infty \exp\left(-\frac{0.693}{T^s_{1/2}(\text{eff})} \cdot t\right) \qquad (B\text{-}3)$$

where F is the fractional uptake by the source organ of the administered activity A_T. $T^s_{1/2}(\text{eff})$ is the time it takes the initially deposited activity to be reduced to half its original value. If the physical half-life is $T_{1/2}(\text{physical})$ and the biologic half-life is $T_{1/2}(\text{biologic})$, the effective half-life of the radionuclide in source organ s is

$$T^s_{1/2}(\text{eff}) = \frac{T_{1/2}(\text{physical}) \cdot T_{1/2}(\text{biologic})}{T_{1/2}(\text{physical}) + T_{1/2}(\text{biologic})} \qquad (B\text{-}4)$$

$\tilde{A}_s$ in this case is given by

$$\tilde{A}_s = 1.44 \cdot F \cdot A_T \cdot T^s_{1/2}(\text{eff}) \qquad (B\text{-}5)$$

Equation B-1 may be rewritten as

$$D(c \leftarrow s) = \tilde{A}_s \cdot S(c \leftarrow s) \qquad (B\text{-}6)$$

where

$$S(c \leftarrow s) = \frac{\sum_i \Delta_i \phi_i(c \leftarrow s)}{m_c} \qquad (B\text{-}7)$$

This term is called the *S-factor* and is the average absorbed dose to the conceptus per unit cumulated activity in organ s. It is commonly expressed in units of rad/(μCi · hr) or Gy/(Bq · s).

Again, it is not practical to try to determine $S(c \leftarrow s)$ for each individual patient and organ. Much data on S-factors are available for radionuclides used in nuclear studies (Kereiakes and Rosenstein, 1980; Snyder et al, 1975; Smith and Warner, 1976). These factors were determined from mathematical computer calculations that assumed a patient of average anatomic proportions.

The total dose, D_T, to the conceptus is obtained by summing $D(c \leftarrow s)$ for all source organs within the mother and within the conceptus that have significant uptake of radioactivity:

$$D_T = \sum_s D(c \leftarrow s) \tag{B-8}$$

This may be separated into two sources of dose:

$$D_T = \sum_{Mo} D(c \leftarrow Mo) + \sum_{co} D(c \leftarrow co) \tag{B-9}$$

Where $D(c \leftarrow Mo)$ is the photon dose to the conceptus from radioactivity in maternal organs (there is no beta dose since electrons cannot penetrate tissues separating the unborn child from maternal organs), and $D(c \leftarrow co)$ is the dose to the conceptus from all radiations originating from within conceptus organs. Equation B-9 may be reduced to

$$D_T = \sum_{Mo} \tilde{A}_{Mo} S(c \leftarrow Mo) + \sum_{co} \tilde{A}_{co} S(c \leftarrow co) \tag{B-10}$$

Smith and Warner (1976) provide S-factors for various radionuclides located in maternal organs of a standard 70-kg adult and assuming a 9.2-mg conceptus. They also provide an S-factor labeled *total body*. This factor applies to activity uniformly distributed throughout the maternal body and the conceptus. It includes the dose from the radioactivity in the conceptus, assuming the activity is uniformly distributed at the same concentration throughout the maternal body. The bladder dose was calculated using assumptions appearing in MIRD (1975a, 1975b, 1976). S-factors for other radionuclides are summarized in Kereiakes and Rosenstein (1980, Tables 29 to 66) and Snyder and associates (1975). These latter data apply only to the nongravida uterus, but they may be used to estimate dose in early pregnancy.

To further simplify dose calculation in some cases, Equation B-10 can be rewritten

$$D_T = A_T \left[\sum_{Mo} \frac{\tilde{A}_{Mo} S(c \leftarrow Mo)}{A_T} + \sum_{co} \frac{\tilde{A}_{co} S(c \leftarrow co)}{A_T} \right] \tag{B-11}$$

or simply

$$D_T = A_T \cdot G \qquad\qquad (B\text{-}12)$$

where A_T is the total activity administered to the mother and G is the bracketed term in Equation B-11.

Several authors have used various data and assumptions to estimate the quantity G. This is the conceptus dose per unit maternally administered activity and is given in Table 3-5 for some radiopharmaceuticals. The dose is obtained simply by multiplying the appropriate table entry by the administered activity measured in millicurie.

Notes on Uncertainties

A major source of uncertainty in these calculations is the determination of the parameter $\tilde{A}_s$. This is particularly true for radionuclides in the bladder and those that cross the placenta. The proximity of the bladder to the uterus makes uncertainties in $\tilde{A}_{bladder}$ critical to accurate calculations. For radionuclides that enter or cross the placenta, particulate radiation will significantly contribute to the dose to the conceptus. This is because the particulate radiation deposits all its energy into the tissues from which it is emitted. For very early pregnancy, a common assumption is that the concentration of the radionuclide within the conceptus is the same as that within the total body of the mother.

Uncertainty in $S(c \leftarrow s)$ stems from two factors. The first is that $S(c \leftarrow s)$ applies to a standard-size woman. The estimate of $S(c \leftarrow s)$ is accurate only insofar as the patient in question resembles this standard patient. The second source of inaccuracy is in Equation B-7. Rao and co-workers (1983) have shown that if the radionuclide is taken up intracellularly, some atomic electron emissions (Coster–Kronig electrons) that are not normally included in the summation of Equation B-7 become important. This is the case, for example, with testicular dose from thallium 201. So if the radionuclide is intracellularly incorporated into the conceptus, these emissions may contribute to a higher dose than anticipated.

Example B-1

Calculate conceptus dose (less than 6 weeks gestation) for an administered activity of 10 mCi of ^{99m}Tc pertechnetate.

From Table 3-5, the dose per mCi of ^{99m}Tc pertechnetate is estimated to range from 0.027 rad/mCi to 0.32 rad/mCi. The conceptus dose is therefore between 0.27 rad and 3.2 rad for the 10 mCi administered activity.

Some of these estimates account for placental transfer of this radiopharmaceutical by extrapolating from data in rats. These estimates range from 0.48 rad to 3.2 rad for 10 mCi. The higher estimates are probably excessive because the extrapolation used has dubious validity. The best estimate is that the dose is less than 3.2 rad, and could have been much lower (less than 1.5 rad).

Example B-2

A patient who received a 2-mCi ^{201}thallous chloride study is discovered to have been about 4 weeks pregnant at the time. Estimate the conceptus dose.

SOLUTION A

From product information on the manufacturer's package insert, the absorbed dose to the ovaries is about 0.5 rad per 1-mCi administration. Very little of this radionuclide is excreted through the bladder (Atkins et al, 1977), and so there is no significant contribution of bladder dose to increase this estimate. A reasonable estimate of conceptus dose is

$$D_T = 2.0 \text{ mCi} \cdot 0.5 \frac{\text{rad}}{\text{mCi}}$$

$$\boxed{D_T = 1.0 \text{ rad}}$$

SOLUTION B

From Atkins and associates (1977), shortly after injection the radioactivity is distributed as follows:

Organ	Fraction of Total Activity
Bladder (urine)	0.04 (after first 24 hours)
Chest	0.10
Kidneys	0.03
Gut and pelvis (lower large intestine)	0.40
Limbs	0.40
Head	0.05
Neck and thyroid	0.01

Assumed similar to body muscle { Limbs, Head, Neck and thyroid } 0.46

This adds up to 103% of the total activity. It is close enough for a reasonable estimate.

The whole-body retention of this radionuclide is such that little activity appears in the urine. As a reasonable estimate, the effective half-life in the bladder, $T^{bladder}_{1/2\,(eff),}$ is assigned a value of 8 hours. For all other organs the $T_{1/2}$ (biologic) is about 10 days. The physical half-life is about 3 days (73.5 hours) (see Appendix C). From Equation B-4, the $T_{1/2}$(eff) is about 56 hours. From Equation B-5:

$$
\begin{aligned}
\tilde{A}_{bladder} &= 1.44 \cdot 8\ h \cdot 0.04 \cdot 2000\ \mu Ci &= 9.22 \times 10^2 \mu Ci \cdot h \\
\tilde{A}_{chest} &= 1.44 \cdot 56\ h \cdot 0.10 \cdot 2000\ \mu Ci &= 1.61 \times 10^4\ \mu Ci \cdot h \\
\tilde{A}_{kidneys} &= 1.44 \cdot 56\ h \cdot 0.03 \cdot 2000\ \mu Ci &= 4.84 \times 10^3\ \mu Ci \cdot h \\
\tilde{A}_{lower\ large\ intestine} &= 1.44 \cdot 56\ h \cdot 0.40 \cdot 2000\ \mu Ci &= 6.45 \times 10^4\ \mu Ci \cdot h \\
\tilde{A}_{muscle} &= 1.44 \cdot 56\ h \cdot 0.46 \cdot 2000\ \mu Ci &= 7.42 \times 10^4 \mu Ci \cdot h
\end{aligned}
$$

S-factors for this radionuclide are (Snyder et al, 1975)

S(uterus ← bladder)	$= 1.4 \times 10^{-5}$ rad/(μCi · h)
S(uterus ← chest [lungs])	$= 4.5 \times 10^{-8}$ rad/(μCi · h)
S(uterus ← kidneys)	$= 5.0 \times 10^{-7}$ rad/(μCi · h)
S(uterus ← lower large intestine)	$= 5.7 \times 10^{-6}$ rad/(μCi · h)
S(uterus ← muscle)	$= 2.0 \times 10^{-6}$ rad/(μCi · h)

From Equations B-6 and B-8:

$$
\begin{aligned}
D_T = &\ 9.22 \times 10^2 \cdot 1.4 \times 10^{-5} + 1.61 \times 10^4 \cdot 4.5 \times 10^{-8} + 4.84 \times \\
&\ 10^3 \cdot 5.0 \times 10^{-7} + 6.45 \times 10^4 \cdot 5.7 \times 10^{-6} + 7.42 \times 10^4 \cdot \\
&\ 2.0 \times 10^{-6}\ rad
\end{aligned}
$$

$$
\boxed{D_T = 0.53\ rad}
$$

This dose estimate assumes no uptake in the conceptus. There are no data available regarding possible placental transfer of this potassium analog.

References

Atkins HL, Budinger TF, Lebowitz E: Thallium-201 for medical use. Part 3: Human distribution and physical imaging properties. J Nucl Med 18:133, 1977

Berman M: Kinetic Models for Absorbed Dose Calculations. New York, Society of Nuclear Medicine, 1977

Dillman LT, Von der Lage FC: Radionuclide Decay Schemes and Nuclear Parameters for Use in Radiation-Dose Estimation. New York, Society of Nuclear Medicine, 1975

Ellett WH, Humes RM: Absorbed Fractions for Small Volumes Containing Proton Emitting Radioactivity. New York, Society of Nuclear Medicine, 1971

Gillespie EC: Principles of uterine growth in pregnancy. Am J Obstet Gynecol 59:949, 1950

Kereiakes JG, Rosenstein M: Handbook of Radiation Doses in Nuclear Medicine and Diagnostic X-Ray. Boca Raton, Florida, CRC Press, 1980

Lathrop KA, Johnston RE, Blau M et al: Radiation dose to humans from ^{75}Se-L-Selenomethionine, (Suppl 6) pamphlet 9. New York, Society of Nuclear Medicine, 1972

Loevinger R, Berman M: A Revised Scheme for Calculating the Absorbed Dose from Biologically Distributed Radionuclides, MIRD pamphlet No. 1. New York, Society of Nuclear Medicine, 1976

MIRD (Medical Internal Radiation Dose Committee): Summary of current radiation dose estimates to humans with various liver conditions from ^{99m}Tc-sulfur colloid. J Nucl Med 16:108A–108B, 1975a

MIRD (Medical Internal Radiation Dose Committee): Summary of current radiation dose estimates to humans from ^{123}I, ^{124}I, ^{125}I, ^{126}I, ^{130}I, ^{131}I, ^{132}I as sodium iodide. J Nucl Med 16:857, 1975b

MIRD (Medical Internal Radiation Dose Committee): Summary of current radiation dose estimates to humans from ^{123}I, ^{124}I, ^{126}I, ^{130}I, and ^{131}I as sodium rose bengal. J Nucl Med 16:1214, 1975c

MIRD (Medical Internal Radiation Dose Committee): Summary of current radiation dose estimates to humans from ^{99m}Tc as sodium pertechnetate. J Nucl Med 17:74, 1976

Rao DV, Govelitz GF, Sastry KSR: Radioactivity of thallium-201 in mouse testes: Inadequacy of conventional dosimetry. J Nucl Med 24:145, 1983

Smith EM, Warner GG: Estimates of radiation dose to the embryo from nuclear medicine procedures. J Nucl Med 17:836, 1976

Snyder WS, Ford MR, Warner GG et al: "S," Absorbed Dose per Unit Cumulated Activity for Selected Radionuclides and Organs. New York, Society of Nuclear Medicine, 1975

Snyder WS, Ford MR, Warner GG: Estimates of Specific Absorbed Fractions for Photon Sources Uniformly Distributed in Various Organs of a Heterogeneous Phantom. New York, Society of Nuclear Medicine, 1978

Appendix C
Physical Half-Lives
of Radionuclides Used
in Nuclear Medicine

Radionuclide	Abbreviation	Physical Half-Life	
Carbon 11	^{11}C	20.3	min
Carbon 14	^{14}C	5730	yr
Nitrogen 13	^{13}N	10.0	min
Oxygen 15	^{15}O	2.1	min
Fluorine 18	^{18}F	1.8	h
Phosphorus 32	^{32}P	14.3	d
Chromium 51	^{51}Cr	27.7	d
Iron 52	^{52}Fe	8.3	h
Iron 59	^{59}Fe	45	d
Cobalt 57	^{57}Co	270	d
Cobalt 58	^{58}Co	71.3	d
Gallium 67	^{67}Ga	3.3	d
Selenium 75	^{75}Se	120	d
Technetium 99m	^{99m}Tc	6.0	h
Indium 111	^{111}In	2.8	d
Indium 113m	^{113m}In	1.7	h
Iodine 123	^{123}I	13	h
Iodine 125	^{125}I	60.2	d
Iodine 131	^{131}I	8.1	d
Xenon 127	^{127}Xe	36.4	d
Xenon 133	^{133}Xe	5.31	d
Ytterbium 169	^{169}Yb	32	d
Thallium 201	^{201}Tl	3.1	d

Index

179